"As people read this book, they will be inspired to know that they are NOT ALONE---and those struggling with eating disorders definitely need to hear that. I am blessed to be a part of this truly amazing project."— **Regina Edgar, 20, United States**

"If you have ever felt like the only one out there struggling with an eating disorder, this book will show you very clearly that you are not. A collection of stories, poetry and artwork by those who are facing the same demons, let this book inspire you to reach out to others and share your story as well. Now you KNOW you are not alone."— **Christina, 24, the Netherlands**

"I really believe in this project, and I'm very grateful to have been given a chance to be a part of it. There are so many real people without a voice and without hope. I think this book can really give them that."— **Katherine Roemer, 19, United States**

"I am sure this book will provide much needed support and help for sufferers of these misunderstood disorders. It is always important to show that recovery is possible and that eating disorders can be beaten." — **Anna Paterson, 37, England**

"I am so excited to be part of this project, and to have the opportunity to share with others the beauty of life in recovery." — **Amanda Travers Bell, 21, United States**

"As in any battle you need to gather as many soldiers as possible to fight with you. A huge part of my recovery success has been due to my boyfriend, therapist, friends & those of you like me. You taught me to find & use my inner voice and now it speaks louder than all the negative voices that the eating disorder had. You are not alone. This book, if nothing else, should teach you that."— **Julie Ramirez, 35, United States**

"I feel honoured to be a part of this project. Never give up; WE all deserve to be happy, healthy and eating disorder free. You can do it!"— **Kim Ratcliffe, 44, Canada**

"I am honored to be a part of this project, I can only hope this book will reach sufferers and their friends and families to let them know they are not alone, and all is not hopeless!" — **Jessica, 26, United States**

"I very much believe in giving people inspiration to continue with recovery, as I know how hard it sometimes feels when you are trying but some days it feels like you are going backwards rather than forward. I want to spread hope that recovery is possible as I can recall very vividly when I was ill that I thought I would never get better and that is why I really believe that this book will be a saving grace for so many sufferers and their families."— **Nadia Lovell, 29, England**

"It has been a blessing to be a part of this book. I pray that it will impact and inspire those who are struggling with eating disorders like so many others encouraged us as we searched for recovery. This book may be the beginning to a deeper understanding and fight for recovery for many struggling women."— **Jessica Beal, 20, United States**

"Thank you so much for giving me the opportunity to contribute to others, it means so much to me. I feel honored to share my story, to let other women know they aren't alone in their struggle and yes, that there is light! Thank you Andrea for making it possible!!"— **Michelle, 31, Canada**

You Are
Not Alone

The Book Of Companionship
For Women Struggling
With Eating Disorders

A Collection of Inspiring Stories,
Poems and Artwork
from 34 Amazing Women
Affected by Eating Disorders.

www.youarenotalonebook.com

ANDREA ROE

TRAFFORD

USA • Canada • UK • Ireland

Note for Librarians: A cataloguing record for this book is available from Library and Archives Canada
at www.collectionscanada.ca/amicus/index-e.html
ISBN 1-4120-9617-0

Printed in Victoria, BC, Canada. Printed on paper with minimum 30% recycled fibre.
Trafford's print shop runs on "green energy" from solar, wind and other environmentally-friendly power sources.

TRAFFORD
PUBLISHING™

Offices in Canada, USA, Ireland and UK

Book sales for North America and international:
Trafford Publishing, 6E–2333 Government St.,
Victoria, BC V8T 4P4 CANADA
phone 250 383 6864 (toll-free 1 888 232 4444)
fax 250 383 6804; email to orders@trafford.com
Book sales in Europe:
Trafford Publishing (UK) Limited, 9 Park End Street, 2nd Floor
Oxford, UK OX1 1HH UNITED KINGDOM
phone +44 (0)1865 722 113 (local rate 0845 230 9601)
facsimile +44 (0)1865 722 868; info.uk@trafford.com
Order online at:
trafford.com/06-1373

10 9 8 7 6 5 4 3 2

Dedicated to all those suffering with an eating disorder,
and the loved ones who support them.

Dear Jocelyn,

It's an honour for me to be in touch with you. You are an inspiration and I'd like to thank you for sharing your story. You are doing an amazing job in spreading the word that recovery IS possible! Love,

Andrea

Trigger Warning!

Please note that the content in this book may trouble some people.

It contains detailed stories of people struggling with Anorexia, Bulimia, Binge Eating, Sexual Abuse, Rape, Physical and Emotional Abuse, Mental Disorders, Self-Harm and other Addictions.

If you feel you may react negatively to the content, please don't continue reading.

Contents

Acknowledgements

It is a real pleasure for me to acknowledge all the wonderful women who have helped me put this book together by donating not only their stories, poems and paintings, but by giving their time, hearts and souls as well. I appreciate all your help very much! Without you, this project wouldn't have been possible!

I'd also like to thank you for the trust that you put in me, for believing in me and my project from day one. I am honoured and proud to have gotten to know you all and I very much enjoyed working together with you. You are very inspiring women and truly AMAZING!

A great big THANK YOU goes to my wonderful family and my amazing husband Brandon for believing in me and always supporting me. Ich hab' euch lieb, Familie! I love you, honey!

I'd also like to thank all my friends in Austria. I know we don't see each other very often anymore, but I want you to know that your friendships are very important to me and that I am very happy and proud to have you in my life!

Last but not least, I want to say 'Thank You" to all the wonderful people I met at and through Landmark Education. Thanks for supporting me and showing me what is possible.

Introduction

RECOVERY IS POSSIBLE

A few years ago I would have never have imagined I would be where I am today. I am a confident woman. I smile and laugh a lot. I love my life! And most importantly, I love myself! I have finally become friends with the person I see when I look in the mirror.

During my eating disorder, I often found it helpful to read stories and poems of former sufferers who had felt just like me but who managed to recover. Their writings gave me strength and showed me that I was NOT alone. I loved reading about other people's eating disorder experiences, recovery and healing journeys. They gave me hope, comfort and much needed support. I felt understood.

Now that I am recovered myself, I see it as a mission to be the one who provides support for those still suffering. I want to share my story and show you that you are not alone, that there is help, there is hope and that recovery IS possible – ESPECIALLY FOR YOU!

In this book you will find personal stories, poems and paintings of women who have not only survived eating disorders, but also depression, social anxiety, self-harm, suicidal thoughts, other addictions, mental disorders, emotional and physical abuse, sexual abuse and rape.

Read this book however you want to – from the beginning to the end or jumping around. See it as your personal portable support group. It is my hope that you read it over and over, whenever you need hope, comfort or support.

My co-authors and I all came together for this project to unite our voices and speak out because we want YOU to know that YOU ARE NOT ALONE! We want you to know that no matter where you are right now – this is not the end. You can get through this! Please don't give up on yourself! Keep on believing in yourself and continue to be strong!

All the best to you from my heart and lots of strength!

Andrea Roe

Please feel free to get in touch with me! Let me know how this book affected you; share your thoughts and stories with me. Feel free to contact me any time with questions, comments or for some support at andrea@eating-disorder-information.com. I always welcome your e-mails!

For more information about the book, or to get a poster of the book cover, please visit www.youarenotalonebook.com. This website also features a 'You Are Not Alone' Forum – a place for everyone with any type of eating disorder who wants to interact with others to ask questions, share experiences, receive and provide support, and talk about emotions and issues surrounding the battle and recovery from eating disorders.

Inspiring Stories, Poems and Artwork

THIS BODY

I am sorry for all the pain I have caused,
for all those knives I have stabbed you with.

I am sorry for all the times I have beaten you up,
for every time I have bruised you and made you sick.

I am sorry for hating you without reason,
for hiding you,
for flaunting you,
for making you feel worthless.

I am trying so hard to treat you well,
but I just cannot seem to get it right.

Yet you stand by me everyday,
giving me life and supporting me,
never judging me,
and even after all the wounds I have inflicted
you are still always there for me.
Please forgive me.

By Lori Henry, 24. Vancouver, British Columbia, Canada. Bulimic for 5 years. Recovered. Author of "Silent Screams", a collection of poems at the core of her journey in recovering from bulimia. For more information, please go to **www. trafford.com/robots/02-0694.html and http://eatingdisorders.suite101.com.**

SUNLESS VOID

I am sitting here in my heart of darkness.
I feel so small compared to the heavy black fog surrounding me;
it is the ugliest void I could ever create,
yet it is mine.
As I sit within it,
calmly and serenely,
the darkness does not lift
but the light seeps in;
and it does not seem so hideous anymore
and it does not look so loathsome.
It is my heart,
It is my soul.
It is me.
And I will not be ashamed.

By Lori Henry, 24. Vancouver, British Columbia, Canada. Bulimic for 5 years. Recovered. Author of "Silent Screams", a collection of poems at the core of her journey in recovering from bulimia. For more information, please go to **www. trafford.com/robots/02-0694.html and http://eatingdisorders.suite101.com.**

My Story

By Anna Paterson, 37. England. Engaged to Simon Teff. Author of Eating Disorder Recovery Books. Anorexia for 14 years. Sexual, Emotional and Physical Abuse Survivor. Self-Harm. Recovered.

From the age of three, I was mentally and sometimes physically abused by my Grandmother. She treated me badly in many different ways, repeatedly telling me that I was worthless, unlovable, ugly and fat even though I was none of these. She constantly played cruel tricks on me (such as force feeding me and abandoning me in shops) and gradually my self-esteem was destroyed. Many horrific memories remain, including the time when I was seven years old and my Grandmother forced me to walk through the Chamber of Horrors in Madame Tussauds. She told me that I was a revolting person and belonged in this place with all the other disfigured and damaged faces.

I saw my Grandmother every day in an attempt to protect my Mother. My Mother suffered from migraines and I realised that these headaches became worse whenever my Grandmother treated her badly. Quickly I learned that I could stop my Grandmother from being cruel to my Mother if I took all the abuse instead. I was too frightened to ever tell my parents about my Grandmother's ill treatment because she said that she would kill my parents if I spoke out about it, so I stayed quiet.

My Grandmother often told me that I was a failure and said that I would never do well at school. This caused me to work even harder at my studies and I would always complete my homework the night it was set. Even though my Gran didn't live with us, she was often in the kitchen with my Mother when I returned from school and I became afraid of going home. I began to join in all the after-school activities available, including swimming, hockey, computer studies and gymnastics. I was wearing myself out though and by the age of 13, my body was no longer able to cope with all the abuse and hard work and it began to shut down.

I developed 'glandular fever' and after many months of illness was admitted to the children's ward of our local hospital. My Grandmother visited me every day and continued to whisper cruel words to me. At the same time, she told the doctors and nurses that she believed my parents were abusing me. The doctors decided to stop my parents from visiting so frequently and instead encouraged my Gran to visit more often. I became very unhappy and stopped eating, so the doctors prescribed adult doses of anti-depressant drugs.

Almost immediately, these powerful drugs caused me to start hallucinating. The doctors thought I was telling them lies to avoid doing my homework and just increased the dosage of the pills. The hallucinations became more frequent and I couldn't look at a page or blank wall without horrific images appearing before my eyes. A few days later another problem developed and I found that I was losing the ability to read and write. When I looked at a page of writing, the words began to swim and move around so that sentences became meaningless.

It took my parents a number of days to convince the doctors that I was telling the truth about my condition and the pills were stopped but the damage had already been done. After I left the hospital, I slowly taught myself to read again with the help of a piece of card that isolated just a few words at a time. Over the next two years I became used to reading and writing in this way and took all my 'O' level classes during this period. It wasn't until I began my 'A' level studies that I was able to read and write normally again.

By the time I was 17 we were having serious family problems. To help with her migraines, my Mother had been on tranquilizers since I was six years old. Now, 11 years later, she was taking a massive cocktail of them together with some very strong painkillers. She had disappeared into her own fantasy world and was writing strange poetry and letters to the singer John Denver. My Grandmother told me that my parents' marriage was in trouble and that they were going to get divorced. She said that this was all my fault.

It was then that I decided I had to disappear. I felt worthless and as if all I did was cause problems. I believed that I no longer deserved food and so stopped eating. I didn't feel this was enough punishment though and also began to seriously self-harm. Trapped in an impossible situation, I realised I was developing anorexia.

For the next four years my weight slowly dropped. I managed to keep my illness under control while my life was relatively calm but as soon as there was any extra stress, that dormant monster anorexia reared its head again. I left college at 19 because I was bullied by a 'friend' and instead started work in a solicitors' office. The first three months were fine but in time my boss began to treat me badly. My Gran's treatment had led me to believe that I deserved to be abused by anyone and he soon realised he could sexually harass and humiliate me. This behaviour continued for over two years.

By the age of 21 I was very ill. Two days after my twenty-first birthday, my parents told me that I was ruining their lives and making them both ill. The guilt

I felt was tremendous but I simply couldn't eat, even for them. I felt totally controlled by an anorexic 'voice' in my head that sounded just like my Grandmother. It told me I was fat and ugly and had to starve myself. It yelled loudly every time I ate, repeatedly telling me I was a very bad person. I was now completely obsessed with food and did everything possible to avoid eating. Unable to force myself to eat, I grew extremely weak and had to give up my job as a legal secretary.

My parents took me to our family doctor who was horrified by my weight loss and immediately sent me to see a psychiatrist at our local hospital. She diagnosed anorexia nervosa and I felt as if my deepest darkest secret had been discovered. I felt ashamed and very alone. I had to agree to see a psychiatric nurse once a week but the shame I felt left me unable to share my true thoughts and feelings with her. Misled by my confusing answers to her questions, the nurse disagreed with the original diagnosis and started to treat me for the illness M.E. (chronic fatigue syndrome).

Relieved that the nurse no longer believed that I was suffering from anorexia, I fell even deeper into the illness becoming more withdrawn every day. Just after Christmas I felt so desperate and alone that I attempted suicide. Halfway through the attempt, I realised that my Mother would return home to find my dead body and I just couldn't hurt her in that way. I felt that I had already caused her enough pain by what I believed to be my 'selfish' behaviour. I put away the knife and bandaged my bleeding wrist.

Later that year, my Father retired from his job and we all moved to Cornwall to try and escape from my Grandmother. I managed to avoid doctors for three months but eventually we had to join the local health centre. The doctor I saw was horrified by my condition. During my physical examination, the nurse had discovered that I was trying to cheat the scales and they realised that my weight was now at a life-threatening level.

After just three months in my new home, I was confronted by two doctors who wanted to admit me to hospital. I tried to beg them to allow me to stay at home but my Mother said that she could no longer cope and I was admitted to my first psychiatric hospital. I was put on complete bed rest because my weight was so low that the doctors were scared that I could have a heart attack at any time. I should have been safe in the hospital but my Grandmother still managed to reach me there. She sent me letters telling me that my parents did not love me and asking why I didn't just let myself die? Instead of showing the doctors this evidence of her abuse, just as my Gran had instructed, I carefully tore up the letters and hid them at the bottom of my waste bin.

After a month, I had gained six pounds and managed to convince the doctors to discharge me. I began weekly therapy that increased to daily therapy as my weight slowly began to fall again. I had left the hospital determined that the anorexia would never win again but after a few weeks at home, it had regained control and the 'voice' was louder than ever. I was once again lying and cheating so that I could lose weight. I hated myself every time I pretended I'd eaten or hidden some food but I felt I had to obey that 'voice'. My parents tried to force me to eat more but this just led me to become even more cunning and secretive.

One horrific day, two years after my release from hospital, I managed to totally block the drainage system in our Cornish home. I can still remember the complete terror I felt when I heard my Father's words: "She's really done it this time! I don't want to call her my daughter any longer!" My Mother was equally angry and said that she didn't believe my Father would ever forgive me. I vowed never to hide food or cheat the scales again but anorexia is a very powerful illness and that whispering 'voice' in my head soon took back control.

Three years after the first hospital admission, my weight had dropped to its lowest ever. I was seeing a psychiatric nurse every day and he was measuring out tiny portions of food for me to eat but my body could no longer process solid food. Even though I was eating, I was losing more weight every day. I tried to fool the doctors into believing I was heavier than I really was but eventually my tricks were discovered and I found myself back in hospital again. This time I was admitted to an eating disorders unit 200 miles from my home, where I was told that I was now just hours away from death.

Looking in the bathroom mirror for the first time since my illness had begun; I saw how I really looked. I was a walking skeleton, with my skin stretched tight over bones. My face had become a skull and when I smiled, it looked like I was wearing a horror mask. For that brief period of time I could understand why everyone was so worried.

The hospital saved my life and I stayed there for six months, working hard at therapy sessions each day. I wasn't completely honest with the doctors though, as the anorexic 'voice' in my head was still very powerful. I had learned so much therapy over the years that I was just repeating it back to them without feeling anything. My occupational therapist did realise what I was doing though and decided to play me the REM song "Everybody Hurts". As I heard the lyrics about holding on and never giving up, I broke down for the first time and started to talk very vaguely about my Grandmother's abuse. When I was discharged from the hospital a few months later, I was physically better but mentally and emotionally I was still very ill.

For the next five years, I lived at home with my parents. The confidence I had developed in hospital slowly began to disappear. I had been able to talk and joke with anyone in the hospital but once I was home, I started to hide in my anorexic shell again. Gradually my weight dropped once more, although I managed to maintain it at a level just high enough to keep me out of hospital. I started my own needlework business but this just gave me another safe reason to stay hidden at home. I led a very isolated life, seeing only my therapists. The few times I went out were with my parents and we lived a very controlled, timetabled existence. I was an adult woman, living the life of a child.

At the age of 29 I felt that my life would never change. I believed that I would always have anorexia and although it stopped me from doing so much, I could see no other options. The loneliness eventually became too much to bear and I joined a pen pal club. Through this group I met Simon, who I soon learned also suffered from low self-esteem. For the first time in my life, I felt able to tell someone about the abuse and my anorexia. This was the real start of my recovery because Simon was able to show me that I was not the terrible person my Grandmother had always told me I was. Slowly I began to realise that I did not need to punish myself by starvation and self-harming. I learned to trust Simon's view of my body rather than my own distorted anorexic view.

Simon was the first person to show me unconditional love and after a few months, we became engaged. With Simon's help, my recovery continued and I am now living a fulfilled happy and healthy life. Recovery is not easy or quick and the fact that Simon was willing to stand by me however long this took gave me the courage I needed to keep making progress.

I decided to share my experiences in the hope that I could help other sufferers beat their eating disorders. I wrote my autobiography "Anorexic" and soon found that many people began writing to me to share their own experiences. I began to realise just how huge a problem eating disorders really were and how little practical information and advice there was available. This is was why I wrote "Diet Of Despair", a self-help book for sufferers and their families. I have since also written "Running On Empty", a novel for young people about eating disorders and friendship. My latest book is "Fit To Die", which is a self-help book that deals with the growing problem of men and eating disorders. I am currently working on two new books - a workbook for eating disorder sufferers called "Beating Eating Disorders Step By Step" and a novel for young people about bullying, "Just Like Doris Day" - they will be published shortly. Through my books, I hope that I will be able to help sufferers and their friends and families to fight these killer diseases. If you would like to contact me, my e-address is Anna@anorectic.fsnet.co.uk and my website is www.annapaterson.com.

By Anna Paterson, 37. England. Engaged to Simon Teff. Author of Eating Disorder Recovery Books. Anorexia for 14 years. Sexual, Emotional and Physical Abuse Survivor. Self-Harm. Recovered. For more information, visit Anna's website at **www.annapaterson.com** or send her an e-mail at **Anna@anorectic.fsnet.co.uk**

My Story and Recovery with an Eating Disorder

By Geri Karlstrom, 53. Surrey, British Columbia, Canada. Recovering for over 40 years from an Eating Disorder.

Eating disorders have devastated my life since I went on my first diet at age nine. I believe that child abuse and trauma were partly the cause of my compulsive overeating, bulimia nervosa and binge eating disorders. I hope by sharing my recovery story and music you will find a friend who understands and the courage to reach out for help.

My name is Geri and I'm recovering from an eating disorder. I've been in recovery for over the past twelve years and would like to share the story of my journey with you.

I'm the eldest of four children and I was born on August 19, 1952 in British Columbia, Canada. My father, a retired Baptist minister, is American and my mother, a homemaker, is Canadian. From the day I arrived into this world Mom dressed me up and showed me off with pride. The love of music was an important part of our family and at the age of four I was coaxed into singing in front of the congregation at dad's church. I was a little shy at first but enjoyed the attention. My parents were pleased to have their children perform. In retrospect I think they wished for perfect children and I was only too willing to do everything I could to attain their approval.

When I was five our family moved to Seattle, where my father completed his education. My parents were strict, old-fashioned disciplinarians and truly did their best to protect their children. Unfortunately, no parent can safeguard a child from all the traumatic things that children are exposed to. At eight years of age I believe I suffered a life-altering experience that scarred me emotionally and put me on the path toward my eating disorders.

One day after school my girlfriend Denise didn't meet me for our daily walk home. With good reason. She had been lured into a vacant garage by the local paperboy who attempted to rape her. He was armed with a knife and when she tried to stop him he retaliated by stabbing her over forty times. He then wrapped her lifeless body in old newspapers and set the garage ablaze. Overcome by guilt, he confessed the crime to his father that evening, a chaplain at the college where my Dad attended. The story of Denise's murder made headlines the next day in Seattle. But instead of discussing this incredibly disturbing event with me, my Mom simply handed me a clipping from the front page of the paper. Numb from the shock, I didn't know that it'd be okay for me to ask questions about something that distressed my parents so much. So I was left to myself to cope and comprehend the brutal horror of Denise's death and heal from the loss of a close friend. Needless to say, I didn't cope well and I certainly didn't comprehend. Sometimes the "no talk" rule translates to neglect and subtle child abuse.

My parents had always made a big deal about appearances, applauding the thin and attractive, and shunning those with less than appealing features. In addition, the early messages I received concerning anything sexual being a dirty and disgraceful thing only added to my bewilderment. Had Denise been attacked because she was desirable? In my juvenile mind I reasoned that if I became unattractive by putting on weight I'd be able to protect myself from men and older boys, of whom I was now terrified. But the push-pull world of trying to look perfect to please my Mom and the fear of being noticed by men put me in a terrible state of confusion. At nine years of age I went on my first diet.

My family loved to celebrate with relatives and church friends. The major focal point of these social gatherings was based on food, as alcohol, drugs and gambling were unthinkable in our religious family. Playing cards weren't even allowed in our house. So food became my escape and sugar became my drug of choice to soothe the stress and pain I felt in childhood. I believe this is one of the many factors that contributed to my eating disorders. But all the calories began taking their toll. My folks sent me to various church summer camps over the years and I found it quite difficult to make new friends. After all, I was now the "pudgy kid" and somewhat of an outcast. The extra weight didn't enhance my natural clumsiness either and one summer I nearly fell into a snake pit in the woods. It wasn't long before I spent most of activity time hanging out at the snack shack. Then one year a wonderful thing happened. I was asked to sing with some other children at camp. After we finished, kids came up and congratulated me on my performance. What a relief! Now I had a way to help me make friends and be liked.

Throughout my troubled childhood the one sustaining force in life had become my love of art and music. It was my dream to be a painter and I also studied piano, but all that changed when I saw The Beatles on Ed Sullivan. I just had to have a guitar, even though "evil" rock 'n' roll music wasn't allowed in my parent's home. So I secretly hid one in the basement and began playing and writing songs. I soon realized that I was able to cathartically express my feelings and experiences in this way, and it became a wonderful time in my life. But I had no idea that my eating disorders would all but rob me of this gift in later years.

Eighteen and ill-equipped to make good decisions, I eloped with the first boy that I seriously liked. It was my way of escaping the dominance of my parents and their constant fear that I'd become a pregnant teen, which would've resulted in my father's dismissal from whatever church he was stationed at. But without knowing it I'd simply traded one controlling atmosphere for another. I had married an angry, violent man who ruled with various forms of abuse. When we had children I'd hoped that he would mellow but this was only a fantasy. In reality things only got much worse. Our two sons, the delights of my life, became his punching bags as well. After twelve years of suffering his words and bruises I finally mustered the courage to escape the hellish storm we called home. That day he had been in another rage and kicked our youngest (who was only five) across the living room floor.

So now I had no partner, no job or training and two kids to provide for. But even though we were so poor I still found ways to medicate myself with inappropriate amounts of food. I was in need of comfort and I destructively found it there.

I had made an independent record album in 1980, Geri Baird - "Coolage"- three years prior to the breakup of my marriage. It wasn't very successful but it gave me the opportunity to work with a number of local musicians and be a part of various bands that were spawned from the project. So when I needed to supplement my "single Mom" income I decided to form a rock band, with the objective of playing downtown Vancouver night clubs. As much fun as it was being a singer/musician for a living, it was hardly lucrative. And the seamy world of early '80s lower class clubs and bars was anything but glamorous. I'd never seen things like illicit drugs and underage prostitutes before. But now I was drinking and experimenting with drugs and chatting between music sets with illegally hired 14 year-old strippers, who worked in another area of the club. Memories of singing in Daddy's church faded into a smoke-filled sunset.

I met my future husband, Ben Karlstrom at a rock concert in 1983. Our paths had crossed a few times before in musically related situations but we'd never really spoken to each other much before that night. He asked me out and on our first date we talked at great length about common experiences like our love of music and misadventures with drugs. He was younger than me, but our similarly abusive pasts and desire to make a better life for ourselves seemed to cement the relationship. I guess that's called, "I'm attracted to your dysfunction. I can relate. You're as screwed up as I am". But I was in love with him and still am. (We're coming up on our 20th wedding anniversary!) He was there for me as I began rebuilding my life after I quit abusing drugs and alcohol. It's interesting to note that my physical sobriety concerning those substances slowly led me back onto the path of overeating. I had modified a few behaviors but the toxic emotional turmoil was still in my system. I simply hadn't addressed any of the issues that fed my destructive eating disorder.

We began writing songs together and making demo recordings, but it took several more years before we got a distribution deal and released our CD "Karlstrom". Throughout that time I binged and purged, eating inappropriately to swallow my feelings of shame and using laxatives and diuretics in an attempt to get thin, especially for promotional photo shoots and concerts we played. I had no idea that I'd developed bulimia nervosa. The desired results didn't arrive though and I was overweight, dehydrated and severely depressed. My new husband was obviously aware that something was very wrong but the more involved he got with my eating disorder the worse my bulimia and binge eating disorder became. I stopped song writing, socializing and gave up hope.

Then one day an interesting thing happened. My husband and I saw a re-run of John Bradshaw's "Bradshaw: On The Family" series on PBS. We were stunned to learn about family systems and how we were set up for certain destructive behaviors. It wasn't long before we began seeing therapists and started the painful process of inspecting our damaged psyches. It marked a new beginning, but things got worse before they got better. On July 4, 1995 I bottomed out. I simply could not stop or control my eating disorder. I felt like I was lost at sea emotionally, physically and spiritually. In the middle of the desperation and blackness of that day I somehow recalled John Bradshaw's story of how he had faced his alcoholism with the support of his friends at Alcoholics Anonymous. At that moment I knew that if I didn't go to a 12-step group for my eating disorders I'd lose everything I loved in life or maybe even take my own life. I chose to go to a 12-step group.

The first meeting I attended was terrifying but I sensed right away that I could get help there. All the methods that I'd tried to heal myself and keep myself safe hadn't worked. It was time to try something new. Amazingly, I felt like I had arrived home. A new place where I was loved and accepted unconditionally. I began to study, work and live the 12-step program and lost some weight. Sugar abstinence was of key importance in this progress. I knew I had a sensitivity to everything with sugar in it so I needed to take it out of my diet completely. I could never have been able to do this without my 12-step program.

I started to feel healthier. Every area of my life seemed to blossom. I began writing songs again and for the first time I was really expressing my deepest feelings in my music. Pain, depression, shame, isolation and despair were changing to happiness, hope, optimism (even during suffering) and a connectedness with others.

And even though I take an occasional step backward there have been so many forward steps that I'm feeling quite secure in this better quality of life. And I'm experiencing greatly improved relationships with my husband, sons and now my parents. The past few years have been an incredible time of healing between my folks and me. The obsession around food issues that has tortured my soul is subsiding and from this newfound peace I'm discovering a place where I'm getting a refreshing new view of the God of my understanding.

I've recorded a number of songs that I wrote over the past four years and compiled them on a CD called Soulful Journey. I feel compelled to give back to the program and people that have helped me so much, so I sing and share my recovery with others in this way. It also helps me in my continuing recovery from my eating disorder. Abstinence has become the most important thing in my life. It gives me back everything I almost lost plus allows me to live a far better quality of life. A world where I can take what I've learned so far and help others by sharing my experience, strength and hope. And that's music to the ears of this recovering food addict.

I CAN'T BELIEVE it's 11 years later from when I started my recovery journey from compulsive eating and bulimia. It's been a struggle with many victories. I can truly say from looking back over the past 11+ years that I've never truly recovered from my eating disorder issues, but there's been steady growth and insight. I realize that this disorder is totally caused by not being able to handle stress in a normal fashion, and by coping with inappropriate food behaviors. When I'm tired, overworked, stressed, angry or even hungry, I find it's a temptation to go back to "cruising the kitchen" for just a little snack to comfort myself.

I've found a few really great behaviors, that when I concentrate on them, work to help me manage my compulsive overeating. I must mention that I simply stopped my bulimic purging 10 years ago when I knew what it was. That's changed for good. I won't abuse laxatives or laxative inducing foods. But what helps me today is that I have a) support friends, b) keep sugar to a minimum in my life, c) have a low carb food plan and d) don't beat myself up for my failures, but accept that this is a life long struggle.

All the best to you and big hugs!

Geri

By Geri Karlstrom, 53. Surrey, British Columbia, Canada. Recovering for over 40 years from an Eating Disorder. Expressing herself through music has helped Geri through her recovery from an eating disorder. If you suffer from eating disorders, abuse, depression or addiction issues, this music is just for you. Geri's music has touched people from all over the world. For more information, visit Geri's website at **www.geri.net**.

SOULFUL JOURNEY

No need to be alone
I sense just how it's going
And I can hear your shame
I know you're lost in blame
Your path will take you
Sometimes to regret
But there's a reason
You'll find your sunset

You're on a soulful journey
Living your one and only life
Yes joy will find you
And love and all that's true

Won't tell you what to do
But I am here for you
You've been hurting for so long
Now it's my turn to be strong
I can't protect you
But I can listen
And I can give you
Some hope you're missing

You're on a soulful journey
Living your one and only life
Yes joy will find you
And love and all that's true
And peace will find you
And hope and all that's true

By Geri Karlstrom, 53. Surrey, British Columbia, Canada. Recovering for over 40 years from an Eating Disorder. Expressing herself through music has helped Geri through her recovery from an eating disorder. If you suffer from eating disorders, abuse, depression or addiction issues, this music is just for you. Geri's music has touched people from all over the world. For more information, visit Geri's website at **www.geri.net**.

COURAGE

In the darkest part of me
Is a deep place I fall
My disease lives in there
I hear the addicts call
So lost in thoughts
And a quest for some relief
Wanting to run from the pain to the peace
But I'll sit with these sorrows
And I'll feel the feelings near
Then I'll learn I won't perish
And find my courage here

By Geri Karlstrom, 53. Surrey, British Columbia, Canada. Recovering for over 40 years from an Eating Disorder. Expressing herself through music has helped Geri through her recovery from an eating disorder. If you suffer from eating disorders, abuse, depression or addiction issues, this music is just for you. Geri's music has touched people from all over the world. For more information, visit Geri's website at **www.geri.net**.

PAINTED DESERT

In the painted desert there's a calm oasis
Where I meet you in the cool of the day
And I hear your voice so soft to me
Saying things are going to be okay
All your worries cares so near just let them go baby
And don't you fear
Keep on trusting keep believing
We're together in the cool of the day

In this painted desert there is sweet assurance
As you're showing me new ways to believe
All the craziness of my troubled past
Fades to nothing in the noonday heat
I see hope in your eyes
Here beneath the blue blue skies
Keep on trusting and keep believing
We're together in the cool of the day

So I come to this place
Where your love has a face
An oasis hidden in the shade
Now my courage is strong
I can keep holding on
I find my solace here in the cool of the day

All your worries cares so near
Just let them go 'cause there's no need to fear
Keep on trusting keep believing
We're together in the cool of the day

So I come to this place where you love has a face
An oasis hidden in the shade

When my courage is gone you say
Keep holding on
A miracle could be only minutes away

By Geri Karlstrom, 53. Surrey, British Columbia, Canada. Recovering for over 40 years from an Eating Disorder. Expressing herself through music has helped Geri through her recovery from an eating disorder. If you suffer from eating disorders, abuse, depression or addiction issues, this music is just for you. Geri's music has touched people from all over the world. For more information, visit Geri's website at **www.geri.net**.

One Life to Live: My Story of Struggle and Victory

By Jessica Beal, 19. United States. Binge Purge Anorexia for 4 years. Self-Harm. Recovered.

My name is Jessica. I am 19 years old and attending Cornerstone University. I am majoring in music performance on saxophone and bassoon. I hope to play professionally in the future and teach college. One thing I have learned throughout my life is that God has been perfectly faithful through both good and bad times. Looking back on my experiences I don't know where I'd be without a Heavenly Father who knows the plans for my life and future. So now I would like to share my story of struggle and victory.

I grew up living a pretty happy childhood, good parents that took care of me and a little brother that became a good friend; but circumstances started to tear down my self worth. I entered high school feeling that I had to earn love by being perfect. I had my music and an immense drive to be perfect. My eating disorders started when I entered High School at 14 years old. I was involved in everything; sports, advanced classes, music in and out of school, lessons, and other activities.

Life soon seemed impossible and out of control. I was stressed out and I was not able to reach that ideal of perfectionism. I also was not very close to my parents at that time. I felt alone and was in search of something to relieve all this stress and to give me some kind of control in my life. I went to a Christian event because I was trying to become closer to God. I knew who He was but I didn't understand His unconditional love and provisions.

Unfortunately my insecurities and my search for something to control made the Christian event that was meant to be good into the thing that would haunt me for the years to come. The event I went to was something called a thirty hour famine. Those thirty hours turned into two weeks for me. By then my parents noticed I was not eating so they made me eat something. I didn't want to because in my head not eating was satisfying and helped me manage the stress of everything. On the day my parents tried to get me to eat I did something I thought I would never do; got rid of my food. I soon realized that purging my food was a lot easier to get away with and keep secret. I thought I had finally found something that would make me happy.

From being around a certain relative of the family I gained a perception that I was never good enough at anything I did and the eating disorder became a way of punishing myself for not being good enough. It also was a way to get rid of stress, hurt and life.

I purged after almost every meal most of my freshmen year. Towards summer I realized I was no longer in control of the one thing I thought I had control over. I needed to stop but I was addicted to it.

Something in me knew that I needed to stop no matter what. Right around that time I read 1 Corinthians 6:19-20. It says, *"Do you not know that your body is a temple of the Holy Spirit, who is in you, whom you have received from God? You are not your own; you were bought at a price. Therefore honor God with your body."*

I held on to this verse and the fact that I didn't want to continue destroying God's temple. I surrounded myself with people that would help and support me so that my decision might be possible. I spent almost every night on the phone with someone, crying because I wanted to purge so badly but I knew I could not give in. I did not stop completely right away but I kept prolonging occurrences and it got easier to not do.

I for the most part was able to stop during the summer. I would mess up once in a while but things were going well. Activities slowed down and life was not as stressful. Then my sophomore year started and so did a million and one activities. I was terrified to start purging again because of how out of control it got last time but I had not resolved the internal issues and I still needed something to relieve all the pain and stress I was feeling. So I started cutting myself. I got deeper and deeper into feelings of hate for myself. I thought I was worthless and that no one cared about me. I had tried multiple times to get rid of the things I used to cut myself but I was too consumed by it to stop. The pain from cutting was much more bearable than the emotional pain. By January 2002 I had plans to kill myself. Luckily a friend realized something was wrong and talked to me, then told my parents. I broke down and cried out to God for help. Since then I have never had another desire to take my life.

Later that year I started restricting food again. I had gained weight and I didn't like it. The eating disorder was now more to lose weight unlike before where it was a punishment and control. I even made it a competition to see how little calories I could eat and how much weight I could lose. During that summer I met the most amazing person. Her name is Minde. It was a miracle that I even met her because there were over 20,000 people gathered at the Alive Christian music festival that day. I thank God that he brought us into each others lives. When I hit the lowest weight I have ever been at she was concerned and traveled out to visit me. She told me I had a problem which I did not believe. I was not throwing-up or cutting. I felt pretty good and I was still eating – but not enough. She began to gain my trust and slowly started to teach me how to eat again. We broke through fear foods, raised my calorie intake and worked through underlying issues. She also helped me to see past all of the lies I had been telling myself for years and helped me to see myself the way God does. What really struck me is that **I'm perfect just the way I am.**

My whole junior year was full of a whole lot of ups and downs. It was discouraging to keep failing at recovery but I knew I had to keep trying. The last time I relapsed was Easter time 2003. I went back to barely eating and exercising excessively. I knew that what I was doing was wrong and I broke down again and cried out to God and was able to finally let go of it. I could not do this to myself any longer. It was not helping and only made me feel worse.

The physical act of eating is now to a point where I can eat normally. I no longer have fear foods or need to count calories and my body has been maintaining at a healthy weight for a year now. After the physical part of me was healed I would still battle internally with thoughts/temptations to go back. Insecurities about who I was, etc.

Through God's word I was able to fight the lies the world and myself had engraved into my mind. **Lies** like *"I'm worthless. No one loves me. I don't look good because I'm not skinny enough, if I loose a few more pounds then everyone will like me more."* **Lies, all lies!** These are lies because no matter how thin I did get I was never happy with myself, I was never satisfied with how I looked. I was not happy until **I learned to accept myself** for the person I am and not worry about what everyone else thinks.

Now in my second year of college God has helped me get to a point where I know there is no turning back. I've found a new joy in life that I didn't know could exist. I will every once in a while have negative thoughts but I've learned to distract myself or pray when those times come. Contrary to popular opinion, someone who struggles with an eating disorder can be completely healed and that is my desire for all of you who can relate to this. I can look in the mirror now and say I am beautiful, I can be happy with who I am and not seek others approval by changing who I am. From where I am at now it is hard to believe that what I just wrote to you was once me. That is why I am writing because there has got to be more to life than living with inner conflict and physical destruction.

As a follow-up, I was in counseling here and there and just did one last year of counseling 2004-2005 to really resolve some things. I never went inpatient or had specific eating disorder treatment. I guess I tell you that because I do not want you to lose hope if you cannot go to counseling but you do need people around you to support and understand what you're going through. I highly encourage counseling if it is in any way possible. So how did I overcome the eating disorder? Countless ups and downs, tears and struggles; but I think what got me through it all was a decision to get better no matter how hard or what happened. **God was always there** with His amazing help and love; so were friends and family who supported me and taught me the truth. ***Please don't give up!!***

Jess

By Jessica Beal, 19. United States. Binge Purge Anorexia for 4 years. Self-Harm. Recovered. For more information, visit Jessica's website "One Life – Sharing, the Key to Hope" at **http://river-tree.net/onelife/**

I AM NOTHING WITHOUT YOU

Lord I trust you, you mean so much to me.
Lord I'm nothing without you
I give you all I say and do.
Lord you're all I want to see
Please close my eyes and mind to the lies that haunt me.
You're the only perfect one,
So perfect I'll never be.
And I'm okay with that.
Lord my body is your temple
And I want to treat it that way
Lord take away the obsession
To need to control how much I weigh.
Lord, I don't know the reasons I do the things I do.
Please make them clear to me
So I can work on them and improve
Until then Lord I offer them all to you.
Lord you said no man can serve two gods
And right now I feel I do.
I'm so concerned about food
That it gets in the way of you.
Lord, I'm sorry for disobeying
And I'm sorry for not trusting you.
You've brought me this far so I know you won't leave
Lord, I give you my life and my body
I give you everything.

By Jessica Beal, 19. United States. Binge Purge Anorexia for 4 years. Self-Harm. Recovered. For more information, visit Jessica's website "One Life – Sharing, the Key to Hope" at **http://river-tree.net/onelife/**

FUTURE?

This world has so much sorrow,
So much stress and so much pain.
It's easy to wonder what we live for.
To wonder why we were made.

You think that you're not good enough,
Like you don't deserve to live.
You think that no one ever loved you,
And that you have nothing to give.

You wander through life confused,
Without somewhere to turn,
You think that leaving is the answer,
The only way out.

You don't see the ones who love you,
The way that they would feel.
To lose a daughter, friend or sister.
A tragedy that can never be repaired.

You can never be replaced in the hearts of the ones who love.
You are you!! Precious, Held and Loved.
You make the world to someone you are Wonderful and Complete.
You can make it in this life just take a look at your feet.

Watch where they take you,
The roads not yet turned,
The discoveries you will make,
and the things that you will learn.

Think about the experiences that lie ahead.
The fun times and beautiful days spent with friends.
Think about your life when you're in college or a mom.
Don't throw so much away even though it seems like the end

Being happy is not impossible.

To love yourself is true,

To keep on going after feeling this way,

Greatly rewards you.

I know from experience that it's not the end.

That everything works out for the best.

That people love you even when you feel the lowest.

That you will be okay.

By Jessica Beal, 19. United States. Binge Purge Anorexia for 4 years. Self-Harm. Recovered. For more information, visit Jessica's website "One Life – Sharing, the Key to Hope" at **http://river-tree.net/onelife/**

The Perfect Girl

By Regina Edgar, 20. Michigan, USA. Anorexia and Bulimia for 9 years. Self-Injury for 5 years. Sexual Abuse. In Recovery.

My name is Regina. I never dreamed that I would be where I am today, and yet, I am here. I am alive. And it is because of this continuation in life that I MUST share my story with you. I believe it is a miracle that I am still living and breathing today, because that life was almost taken from me by a deadly eating disorder.

I grew up in a loving family. My mother is a Christian, but my father remains unsaved. There was always a lot of discord in our family, and my parents fought a lot. But, I was always the peace-maker, and I never made it known that their fighting hurt me too. Many hours I would spend upstairs crying to myself, only to wipe away those tears and put on the smile that everyone loved. I was never a fan of conflict, so I always tried to make everyone happy. I was your typical people-pleaser, all-A student, top "Godly knowledge", an aspiring violinist, and a perfectionist all the way. I learned at an early age to do everything within my power to make others feel good and be happy, and to push my own feelings aside. I never got angry. I programmed myself not to feel that emotion—or any emotion. From the conflict in my family, I learned that emotions only hurt people…and I could not handle getting hurt. So, I dismissed my emotions. Never dealing with them again. My family was very controlling, but only I could control how I felt.

I was always a skinny little girl. I could eat anything, and still be stick-thin. Momma called me "Bean-pole"; Daddy called me "Zipper". I took pride in that thinness for so long. It was my identity. But, around age 11, it took on a whole new meaning for me. I had been hurt by many people, and because of that, I decided never to trust anyone again…and it remained that way for most of my teenage years. My thinness became a quest of destruction, and my body repulsed me. Perhaps it was fueled by my hitting puberty—for I was afraid (and probably still am) to become a woman instead of a little girl. But no matter what all took place to lead me there, I started down a deadly path of anorexia. I found out that even when others controlled everything about me, they could not control my weight or what I ate or didn't eat. I was in control of that—or at least I thought I was. At first,

I would only eat half of my lunch at school. Then, I'd start skipping breakfast. This went on into my teenage years until it got to a point where I weighed less at the age of 14 then I did when I was 11 years old. I no longer ate breakfast ever, I threw away my lunch at school, and I would do my best to eat minimally at dinner time. Often, I would chew my food up at the table, only to spit it into my napkin.

I have always been anemic, but during those years, I became excessively so. I got dizzy all of the time, and blacking-out was a daily occurrence. I passed out or fell down several times, but I always kept that mechanical smile—the smile telling everyone that I was all right.

It was at this age that my young career started blossoming. My violin-playing became the passion of my life even more. I started playing the music of my ancestors, the Irish, and became the fiddler for a Celtic band. I have always been a hard-worker, pushing myself beyond normal limits, but this new-found love fueled this determination even more. I practiced 7-8 hours a day, and loved every minute of it. The band grew, we produced several of our own recordings, and we started playing concerts on stages around our state. I felt amazing. My dreams were coming true…but the eating disorder was still there. With the added pressure of 'stage-appearance' and the added stress, my starving got even worse and I ate even less. I felt I needed to be perfect in all aspects, and that included looking perfect. To me, I never saw what everyone else saw, and when I looked in the mirror I saw nothing but imperfection.

And I remember it clearly now. December 23rd, 2001, my self-hatred and stuffed-pain became too much. That evening, I took out a knife and cut my arm three times. I will never know what possessed me to even think of that, but I felt freedom and release from seeing what I had done. From that moment on, I found out that I could take care of the pain and my perceived imperfection on the inside by making it visible and painful on the outside. And that started my hellish trek into self-injury. My arms became a battlefield of all the pain I could not express emotionally, and day by day I would cut myself, roll down my sleeve, put on the smile hiding what I felt, and I would once again become the 'perfect girl' everyone believed me to be.

After a while of wearing long-sleeves all year-round and wincing in pain whenever anyone touched me, people started questioning me. So, I started being even more secretive and cut on my legs instead. It was at that same time I struggled to hide the fact that I did not eat. People would ask me questions and I would have to eat—just to show them that I was "fine." That's when I found restrictive-bulimia. I felt confident in the fact that I could starve myself, but if anyone ever made me eat, I could always get rid of the food by vomiting. The deception was a huge part of everything. I no longer was myself, but a mask of who I thought everyone wanted me to be. And deep down, behind those smiles, was a girl struggling to survive in her own self-hatred, hidden emotions, and imperfections.

My escape from myself came in three forms: starving, bleeding, or with my head peering into a toilet—a far cry from the confidence I portrayed on stage. I felt so fake—but that is all I knew. The real Regina had been lost since early childhood when she first found out that she would rather hide emotions then feel the pain of life.

I played this deadly game for years, getting sicker and sicker, and losing more and more of myself. However, after an amazing stage performance at the age of 17, my life came to a sudden halt. I was diagnosed with a deadly childhood cancer, and my days were filled with doctor appointments, surgeries, chemotherapy (losing my hair), radiation, sickness, and hospital stays. I thought that I would die, and doctors, family, and friends believed the same. My whole focus shifted to fighting to live, and I believe my faith is the only thing that kept me alive. God held me, protected me, and gave me the grace to be okay with whatever came in the face of the cancer. I grew stronger in Christ, and I was at peace with whatever He brought my way—be it life or death. I knew that God was in control and that He was being glorified through me.

However, even during that time, the eating disorder plagued me. I lost a lot of weight because of treatments, but the anorexic part of me loved it that way. I was not able to eat because of the sickness, so they hooked IV food up to me. I cried in the hospital, logically knowing that that food was saving my life during this cancer, but feeling awful because the eating disorder screamed that I "was not allowed to have any food" and that I would get fat from it—when in reality, I was wasting away into a sickly waif.

After a while, miraculously, the cancer was put in remission and I started to get healthier. I felt it a blessing to even be able to eat without getting sick from chemotherapy, and I thought my worries with the eating disorder were over. After all, I had been given a second chance at life—cancer didn't kill me. I was alive! However, shortly after I was put in remission, the eating disorder picked up exactly where it left off. I had gained weight when my health returned, and the eating disorder would have none of it. So, I fell back into the starving and vomiting. But a new element was added—laxatives. I was determined to get rid of any amount of food I ever had to put into my body. So, not only did I throw up after meals, but I would over-dose on laxatives too. This continued. I graduated from high-school as the valedictorian, and stood among peers and teachers, skirt hanging loosely from my deteriorating frame…thinking that after moving away from home to go to college I'd find a new life and not have so many problems. At least, that is what I hoped.

I moved to college at Cornerstone University, and honestly thought I was doing better. I only ate one meal a day, but I truly thought that that was 'normal' and 'okay'. I thought I was better. I gained weight and I was having fun with friends. I thought I was over any destructive behavior that plagued my past.

It was that first year in college that I met Jessica*. God had a miraculous connection with her and I one evening. She shared her story of her struggling with eating disorders and cutting, and I could not believe my ears. I had never heard of anyone struggling with the same issues that I did. So, I told her my story, as well—and how I was recovering (which I honestly believed at that time). However, that same semester, I found myself cutting again, starving more, and purging.

That continued into the summer of 2005, where everything got extremely worse. I had my own apartment, and I was able to be even more secretive than I was before. The cutting got worse, and I barely ate. My break-time at work was spent vomiting into the toilet of a dirty public restroom—desperate to get rid of the food that my co-workers kindly offered to me to eat. My evenings were spent exercising compulsively and cutting before I went to bed. Jessica called me one evening when I was hurting so badly. I had been throwing up a couple of times each day, and my legs were a bloody mess of scars and cuts. I confided for the first time that I was in trouble. I told Jess what was happening, and how I wanted to be free from all of it. So, over the phone, we communicated and started a plan to help me get better. I started with eating small and trying to keep it down. Together, we kept in touch, and I was able to eat somewhat normal for a couple of weeks—which was a huge accomplishment for me, as I had never eaten that much in years. But then, I panicked—I had no way to cope because eating disorders were the only way I knew how to deal with life. I plummeted. I started restricting, purging, and cutting even more. I had publicity photos taken for my music, and I felt that I looked hideous in them. I needed my control back.

I left for Cornerstone for my second year, and the eating disorder was worse then ever. Those first few weeks I ended up losing quite a bit of weight, and I kept getting worse. Jessica was there with me all the way. She finally came to a point where she told me that I needed more help than she could give me. So, together (with her posing as me on the phone since I was crying too hard to make myself do it), we called our school counseling office and set up an appointment for me. I was scared out of my mind, but I went. It turned out to be amazing, and I truly loved my counselor. I was sent to the school nutritionist from there, only to find out that my blood levels were not where they needed to be. I was in an anabolic stage, which meant that my body was feeding off of itself for a very long time. This scared those around me because no one knew if my body was feeding off of vital organs or not. So, Jess helped me again to start eating a little bit each day, and the nutritionist put me on nutritional supplement drinks to help me get out of the anabolic state. I told my suitemates what was going on, and they helped me as well. However, with the eating getting better, the cutting and purging only got worse. I was cutting deeper and more frequently; I was even starting to scare myself. I bled through a lot of clothes, and walking was a huge task because of the pain I had to disregard as the cuts covered my legs.

Soon after that they sent me to an eating disorder specialist for therapy once a week, but nothing got better. She brought out painful memories that I had suppressed, and it only heightened my desire to destroy myself. I hated how I looked, and I started wearing even bigger clothes than the baggy ones I was shrinking out of. I hated my body and wanted no one to see what I looked like. I despised the face I saw in the mirror.

After about 2 months of trying to eat, I gave up. I could not do it anymore, and the eating disorder fully took over. I stopped eating. I cut multiple times a day, as deep as the strength in my arm would press down. I took laxatives throughout the whole day, and I vomited whenever I was made to eat. I got so weak that walking to classes was a burden. I couldn't even force myself to practice my fiddle. I had lost interest even in the music that gave me so much life before—and that truly scared me. I slept most of the time, for I had no energy to do anything else. I took about three naps a day, and only awoke when my worried suitemates came in to see if I was all right. I secluded myself from everyone, and I found myself getting depressed.

I stopped eating for days in a row, and one morning found my heart racing exceptionally fast. I could barely walk to get into the shower, and kept feeling myself 'start to lose it' and about to faint. It was Sunday, December 4, 2005. I confided in my suitemates how I felt that day, and they in turn told me I needed to get help. We all went and talked to Jessica, and they all basically agreed that I needed further help. They called my counselor, but were disappointed when she told them to wait to see my therapist on Wednesday. I was relieved because I was too scared to get more help. My suitemates and Jessica talked to me and asked questions, but I do not remember much of what they said. All I do know is that every time I spoke, they told me that I wasn't making sense. I wasn't being coherent. The eating disorder had consumed me, and there was nothing rational left within me. All that came out of my mouth was destruction, and I was too blind from the eating disorder to see it. I fought them, because I couldn't make sense of what they were trying to do to me.

Well, Wednesday, December 7th came and I shall never forget that day. Jess went to therapy with me and told my therapist of her concern. By that time I was in another one of my 'starving escapades' and had not eaten much for a couple of days. I was mentally gone, drained. My therapist called around, and with the providence of God found ONE bed in all of the area that was open in the psychiatric hospitals. We believed it a miracle that God allowed a place to be open when it seemed impossible. They held the bed for me, and I cried. I remember crying in Jessica's arms while my therapist set up all of the details. I was literally in hysterics as she held me there. "I don't want to go! I am not sick! Please don't do this to me!" I cried. But, Jessica had the grace of God, and gently held me and told me I'd be all right. I know it was one of the hardest things she had ever done, but her strength covered me when I was a wreck there in that room.

I had about three hours before I was to be at the hospital's office. So, Jessica and my suitemates packed up my belongings and helped me get ready to go. There were many tears and worries as they took me to the psych ward. I felt deserted as I was admitted and separated from my friends. I knew they loved me, but I could not understand why I had to be there and why I could not be with them. I felt alone. I cried for almost 3 days straight as I was in group after group, had blood taken and checked, had many nurses checking on me, weighed every day and not able to see the weight, forced to eat, and monitored at all costs. I felt like a prisoner, and I was scared. I was diagnosed with anorexia, bulimia, self-injury, anxiety, and major depression. They put me on medication.

Over the days spent there, I realized that I was not alone. God was with me—even there in a locked-up hospital, God was there. And, I gradually started to feel, I mean really FEEL. It was scary, because I had never felt like that in my entire life. I felt a tiny bit of 'real-ness' as I sat there trying to eat what they told me to. I had hit rock bottom and I had no where else to go. It was there in a mental health psychiatric ward, that I hit a breaking point and was able to think clearly for the first time in a long while. I realized that God wanted me to get better. There was more to life out there. God had saved me by putting me in that hospital. I know that I would have come closer to death over Christmas break if God had not put those people in my life at that time to get me to that hospital. It was there that I realized for the first time, a little part of me wanted to be FREE for MYSELF. I, Regina, wanted to get better for me. I believed that God had a plan in all of this, and I believed that He would be glorified through me. I realized that it was His strength that had given me life thus far, and only His strength could continue to help me out of this pit.

Every evening in the ward, I would sit at the payphone and talk to Jess. We talked of God, of freedom, of a better life; Of my future—eating disorder-free. I was filled with new ambition and a determination to get better.

Today, I am out of the hospital. Today, I am trying to eat. Today, I am trying to eliminate cutting and today I am not purging. I am now at a healthy weight and I am being monitored by professionals. I go to counseling and therapy still, and have appointments with a dietician and psychiatrist. The depression has gotten better and I am learning to work through my anxiety. I am not wholly better, but I am more stable now than I have ever been. Each day, I struggle with thoughts and desires to go back into my destructive behavior. And, I will not lie—I have had days where I cut myself or do not eat enough, and I constantly look into the mirror and see someone who I do not like. But, this time it is different because I pick myself back up and start anew the next day. This time it does not feel hopeless. I am surrendering all of this to God, and He is guiding me through it. Yes, I fear that I will fall heavily back into that trap. I fear it every time I have a thought, every time I eat, every time I feel like purging, and every time I slip-up and cut, or those times when I do not eat. But, I know that I have God on my side. He is taking care of me. I want to get better for Him and the future that He has for me. I want to glorify Him, and I know that He does not want me to hurt through eating disorders and self-injury.

Each day is a struggle, but I know that I can get better. We all can get better. There is so much to live for.

Regina

By Regina Edgar, 20. Michigan, USA. Anorexia and Bulimia for 9 years. Self-Injury for 5 years. Sexual Abuse. In Recovery. Feel free to contact Regina at **youngfiddler@hotmail.com**.

---

* Jessica's story and poems are also in this book.

THIS IS MY LIFE!

This is <u>my</u> life.

How dare you try to take it from me!

I'm sick of listening to all of your lies.

There's nothing you can say that I will believe.

The harder you push me, the harder I'll try.

I'll be damned if you think I'll lie down and die.

You can do what you want, because I've been through it all.

You may cause me to stumble, you may cause me to fall.

But I'll never give up. I won't stay down.

I'll always get up, 'cause I was lost, but now I'm found.

God showed me the way.   He saved me from you.

Sheltered in His arms, there's nothing you can do.

He has special plans for me and they don't include you.

So just go somewhere else and do what you do.

'Cause I'm stronger than you think and I'm angry inside.

There's a fire within me that grows.

A hate for you that I will not hide.

You've had me long enough, always under your control.

So much of my time wasted, so much pain to my soul.

Now, I'm going my separate way. I'm leaving you behind.

You're everything I don't want to be; you're everything I despise.

I'm tired of all the hell that you've been putting me through.

You don't care about me and I sure don't care about you.

So, just get out of my life, 'cause you're not welcome here.

We're done. We're through

By Jamie Walker, 31. Nebraska, United States. Battling an Eating Disorder and Depression for 13 years. In Recovery. Planning to go back to school later this year and finish getting her Human Services degree.

A Victory over My Struggles with Eating Disorders

By Emma McClelland, 18. Manchester, England. Anorexia for 2 years turned Bulimia for 1 year. Self-Harm. Recovered.

I'm not sure exactly where or how to start telling my story but I know that I don't want it to be negatively triggering to whoever reads it. A lot of true stories that I read make me feel like I "wasn't a good enough anorexic" or they made me want to lose even more weight and destroy myself completely. It's for this reason that I'm not discussing weight at all. Eating disorders aren't primarily about food and weight anyway - they are about you!

At about fourteen, shortly after my granny died, my mum told my younger brother and me that she had been having an affair whilst my dad had gone to work (and live) in Germany for some time. She had fallen in love with someone else. I can't remember how I felt. It seems silly to say that but I just can't. I missed my dad so much when he was living away and he continued living there for a while so that *Tom and I didn't have to see how devastated he was. Tom and I reacted differently to the changes that were starting to happen. While my brother became argumentative I became very inwardly focused and slipped into depression. I can still see myself curled in the corner of my room as it span around me, sobbing and clutching my wrist as blood dribbled down it. Despair was the right word for that time. I kept my self harming quite hidden as I did with the laxative abuse that soon followed.

Then things got worse. My dad was dropping off my brother at his friend's house and he got talking to his mother *Julia (whose daughter was also in my school and in my year). Julia was also divorced and the two of them started seeing each other. My brother was furious and upset - why wouldn't he be? I, meanwhile, became caught up in how fat I looked. I would lie, looking at my stomach for ages, pulling at it and hating myself more and more with every second that passed.

My dad promised my brother that Julia and her children would not move into our house. That was important as it was our childhood home, full of memories that will be forever close to my heart yet forever spoiled. They did move in. My brother was livid and he argued a lot with my dad. I, however, had been swept up in other preoccupations.

Eating disorders, as you might know, are the way of the sub conscious to keep the sufferer so focused inwardly that they can't think or feel other difficult emotions or face up to hurtful things. It provides control, an escape from reality. That is what it provided me with - a way to cope with all of the changes around me. What was I feeling as things around my home transformed - the rooms, the layouts, and most importantly the whole sense of the place, the dynamics changed? Did it ever really hit me that my family had suddenly and from nowhere exploded into a completely different state? Did it hurt that the security and comfort I had had for my whole life was ruined? In one house two families pushed together into one awkward and emotional mess and in the other a confusing new place - not as unbearable as our former house now was but still a little strange and charged with unidentifiable feelings. I had my eating disorder and that was it! That was the meaning of my life. The more weight I lost the happier I felt. I had control of this. I was the one with this power. Julia's daughter could be the 'daughter' of that house now - she could replace me if that was what was going to happen. The memories I had made with my friends she could wash over with her own. I didn't feel anything but a drive to lose weight, avoid food, exercise and hate myself.

So in a disgusting way anorexia helped me to bypass the feelings that I couldn't face up to. I had control of this one thing and it filled me with a sense of pride and joy. Anorexia became a voice in my head. It was a she - a friend.

I don't want to detail too much about the ways I suffered. All I am going to say is that through the school nurse my parents discovered my problems and began pushing me to eat, to gain weight, to see a therapist. There were a lot of arguments. I screamed, my dad shook me and shouted and failed to understand me, my mum weighed me a lot then cried and made me feel guilty each time I had lost weight. My friendships became strained and I drifted from a lot of people. Why would they want to be around a ghost of a girl who loves starving more than her own friends?

People noticed my weight loss. I was not shockingly skinny though. I was on my way there and I was miserable but hated even the thought of reversing my trail towards hospitalization. That was my plan. The thought made me happy and it made me safe. Nobody in day to day life had to hear the screaming and the swearing from my parents though, nobody had to cry hysterically each time food was placed in front of them and nobody saw the way my mother broke down each time the numbers on the scale below me dropped. They will never know the way the cold stung inside my bones and made me feel like I was being stabbed. They won't hear what I heard in my head every single day. It was exhausting. I wanted to give up.

I started going to the gym every day, sometimes twice if I could. I was not eating nothing you must know this. I was eating a little - not enough to keep warm, not enough to have a menstrual cycle (that stopped two years ago and has only returned two months before today as I am writing this), not enough for my kidneys to function properly and so I usually woke up about five or six times during the night. I often spent ten minutes in the afternoon looking at a can of diet pop and debating whether the eight calories in it were worth quenching my thirst! I cried a lot, especially after I was made to eat. Even an apple was a disgusting amount to me. I resented everyone who got in the way of my weight loss. My long term boyfriend couldn't cope with my personality change and on a phone call which will always be the worse in my life, we both cried and it was decided that we had to split. I was devastated. What we had can't be described by some hyperbolic metaphor - we were soul mates. But I had screwed up. Anorexia had managed to suck out the essence of which I was and had left me a hollow shell. That is not who my boyfriend had fallen in love with.

It was then that a part of me lit up - a tiny flicker of resistance that realized how important it is to be me and to be happy. I went to my counseling and it was the second woman I went to see who really helped me.

Even now I still think that she is an angel. With her I worked through my problems without her judging me, guilt tripping me or shouting as other people did. She brought what was really troubling me to my attention and guided me through my recovery, explaining any feelings I experienced that confused or troubled me.

I joined a website - an eating disorders community for people who help each other and support each other in recovery. There I found so much encouragement and made friends who understood what I was going through. The more I posted on there the more I realized that my words to others were applicable to myself.

I wrote diaries to vent my feelings and just kept on pushing through the emotional turmoil of gaining back weight and shaking away the voices that plagued my head.

Recovery comes in fits and starts. There are phases of it and it is very emotional.

I went through a stage of binge eating which distressed me very much. I over ate a lot and started slipping into bulimic habits in tearful attempts to reverse my 'mistakes'.

But I carried on with self persuasion that what I was doing was o.k. Eating was good for me - like medicine that would keep me healthy in the correct dosage. I would tell myself that I was beautiful, sometimes out loud. When I ate I would think, "Its ok, it's going to be alright soon. Keep at it."

Practice makes perfect - the more I pretended to myself that I was confident, body happy and fun, the more like my old self I became. I was taking Prozac and that helped me to feel happier and therefore to eat more. I stayed for a long time at a weight just below medically 'healthy' because I was scared to let go.

It was too frightening for me. I had made so much progress but I couldn't push myself far enough. I was in limbo between unhealthy and healthy. Then one holiday I went away skiing - something that I love to do - with positive, fun people. I had fun, I ate lots and although it hurt to do it, I felt like I could no longer restrict.

"I don't care." I would tell myself. I asserted these three words every time I ate more than I was comfortable with.

It has been a long time - but I have beaten anorexia and bulimia. I suffered for two years. I know that I sill have issues with my appearance and I may always have but I remind myself of what is important to me in my life and I can push the anxieties away. Since recovery I have built back up my social life - people want to be with me, people like the positive, happy vibes I give off and I can laugh and joke with people. I can be proud that the effect I now make on people will be positive - not some strange shy, preoccupied girl who cries a lot and eats a little. I can concentrate, I can achieve things, I have energy to do what I want to do, and I enjoy my food (that is an amazing thing). I can appreciate so much in the places I go and in the things I do. I can go out drinking, dancing and having fun. I can act, sing, ski and write to the best of my ability nowadays. I can be a better friend, lover, daughter, sister - I can be me. And that is the greatest gift in the world.

I know what you are feeling and I know that it is harder than words can possibly express. But I know that you can do it - I know that you can recover. My faith and support is with you. Don't give up.

God Bless.

By Emma McClelland, 18. Manchester, England. Anorexia for 2 years turned Bulimia for 1 year. Self-Harm. Recovered.

---

* Name has been changed to protect person's privacy.

ED

He is always there, watching my every move.
Sometimes he compliments me
and tells me I am beautiful
but only to then whisper
that I will not be beautiful if I eat that.

Sometimes he tells me
I am not good enough,
not pretty enough.
"Your fat" he says.
"You are nothing without me".

He lurks around all the time waiting,
waiting until I am happy and content.
He creeps in slowly to destroy my recovery
and ultimately my happiness.

He wrecks every relationship I have
or even could have with others.
He taints the love and support I feel from them
and tells me I can only recover if I am on my own.

So I push them away and we are alone again.
Sometimes he waits.
A week maybe two, maybe even a month.
Once he waited an entire year.
But he always comes back
and I always let him in
and listen to what he says.

Will he ever go away?
Will I ever be able to breathe easy
and just know that he will never return?
Or will I always need to stay on the lookout?

By Julie Ramirez, 35. United States. Bulimia for 10 years. In Recovery.

Letting Go Of Ed

By Sarah Kipp, 26. Las Vegas, Nevada, USA. EDNOS (Eating Disorder Not Otherwise Specified) for 14 years. In Strong Recovery.

My name is Sarah and I have an eating disorder. I have been diagnosed with what is called EDNOS. That means "eating disorder not otherwise specified". For the past 14 years of my life I have gone between either meticulously restricting, or eating a minimal amount and purging. I used various methods of purging including induced vomiting, laxative abuse, diet pill abuse and over exercising.

I still remember the day I was officially diagnosed with an eating disorder. I had gone through a week of pure hell; running for miles everyday and eating far less calories than I was able to burn off. I found myself on the floor of the restroom at home, after a failed attempt to induce vomiting, shaking and determined to make it work. I was so terrified with my behavior that I went to my doctor and told her what had been going on. Tests revealed significant drops in my protein and potassium levels, I was dehydrated, and all I could think about everyday in life was the number on the scale. My doctor began treating me with anti-depressants and referred me to a counselor.

Through my initial counseling, I found that my eating disorder started nearly 14 years earlier when I was in 6th grade. I can remember thinking how much bigger I was than some of my best friends. I always felt "bigger" and thought I never quite measured up because of my size. My mom sent me to school everyday with a nicely packed lunch, but everyday on my way into the lunchroom I simply threw the bag away and went to play on the playground. I was always a very athletic person, involved in various sports and dance classes from the age of 8. So life kept me very active, however, I still felt huge.

The middle of my eighth grade year proved to be one of the most stressful times in my life. My parents decided to move our family to a new state and I was terrified. I was raised in a fairly large city, and attended the same school district for 7 of my 8 years of school. Now I was forced to start over. In the beginning, I gained quite a bit of weight. However, I quickly realized this could become an amazing opportunity for me. I could completely reinvent myself and start over with a clean slate. This is when things became intense.

At my new school, I had to constantly be involved in sports and activities. I quickly learned how to "diet" and started a new one quite often. I started playing soccer on the city league and was very involved with volleyball, basketball and softball through my church. These crash diets quickly became my downfall because the results were never lasting and I began telling myself I was just a failure. The diets soon turned into a punishment I gave myself for some other failure in life. I was around 15 years old when I started taking diet pills. I remember absolutely begging my doctor to give me the big diet fad at the time. To my disappointment, he told me I was not overweight enough. I actually asked him how much I needed to gain in order to be on the pill. I would have done anything to get it. But it never worked, and I was never prescribed the medication.

Throughout high school things only got worse. I played on the soccer team and heavily restricted through the most rigorous training of the year. At soccer camp I rarely ate, and was constantly fatigued and had a hard time keeping up with the training. A fellow teammate brought my actions to my coach's behavior and I was told I needed to immediately work on this if I wanted to stay on the soccer team. Soccer was my life. All I looked forward to everyday was practice and games. A few weeks later I was pulled into my high school counselor's office. She asked me to sit down and told me that a "concerned" friend came to her worried about my weight and my lack of eating. This, of course, infuriated me. I told the counselor everything was fine and I was only losing weight because of the intense soccer training. For the next several days, I was consumed with finding out who reported me to the counselor. I could not see at the time that they were only trying to help. I never did find out who it was that was concerned enough to talk to the counselor, but I now can see how much courage that took.

After high school, I moved back to my hometown for college. This, again, was quite the transition. I had never lived away from my parents, and in the beginning it was very hard. I gained weight and became extremely depressed about my circumstances. So I did the only thing I knew how to do. I started dieting, and got myself a membership to a gym. This time, the weight came off very quickly. I had a very strict routine that involved very little eating and a lot of exercise. I was always leery about dating because I never felt good enough or pretty enough for anyone. So any relationship was short and I was very detached.

Over the next several years I continued to go downhill. I had a job with crazy hours that allowed little time for sleep. I felt sick all the time for one reason or another, and went through many surgeries ranging from carpal tunnel to the removal of a tumor on my ovary. I started hanging out with different friends, the ones dubbed as the "party group". I began going against my beliefs and upbringing, going out quite often to drink and have fun. I experienced some intense value conflict, but always felt I never deserved any better. I was lying in the bed that I made for myself.

After going through these patterns with my counselor, she pegged me as a perfectionist and concluded that many of my insecurities stemmed from the need to please other people. My adolescent and teenage years were spent being what I thought was the model child. I did well in school, always went to church and gave 110% in everything I did. It seemed everything had suddenly worn me down, and I had no idea what exactly I wanted out of life, outside of everyone else's expectations.

Although I was going through therapy, I continued getting worse as I dealt with my grandmother's terminal illness and death. She was the only grandparent I had ever known, and I made many trips to see her towards the end of her life. It was such a privilege for me to be a part of the process, to help take care of her, and be with her as much as possible. However, I did not realize at the time how bad things were getting. I rarely ate, but when I did I purged everything in me in one way or another.

On one of my weekly visits to my doctor, she told me to go straight home and wait for home health. Apparently my levels were so bad that she needed to give me IV therapy. When the nurses came it took them 8 tries to get the IV in my arm because I was so dehydrated. I spent the next 48 hours stuck in my house getting infused with protein and potassium. It was terribly depressing, yet did not change things.

In yet another attempt to start over, I packed up and moved across the country to live with my brother. This was one of the worse decisions of my life. The depression came on full force, I started experimenting with the laxatives, and they soon became a staple of life. I worked in a restaurant, which was the absolute hardest atmosphere for me to be in. It curbed my appetite even more to serve other people and see them eat food. Food literally became the enemy. I began living on eating very little food. This time I dropped weight so quickly that my hair began to fall out and I started receiving comments from others about how pale and sick I looked. This was devastating. How could I have let it go this far? How had Ed completely taken over my life?

I realized it was time for some serious help. I called around to many treatment centers, but with very limited insurance, I ran into the same response; we can not treat you, but good luck with finding treatment. I talked to many people, called many city offices, trying to find a grant or financial aid of some sort to get myself into treatment, but to no avail. I found myself lost in a new city, far from home, few friends to speak of, and became completely consumed with my eating disorder. I did start attending various EDA (Eating Disorders Anonymous) meetings and found support there, but it just wasn't enough. Everyday was spent thinking of ways to continue in my disease, without suffering the long term effects. I could not remember life without Ed, nor could I imagine it.

The next step was moving back home. I had a strained relationship with my parents because of my ignorant choices over the past few years, and all I wanted was to be close to them again. Life got slightly better being surrounded by familiarities; however Ed still hung on for dear life. I began looking into treatment centers again but continued receiving the same response. Until one day I sent an email to a treatment center in California. I received a very unexpected phone call from a certified eating disorder specialist named Laurie*. This phone call changed my life.

Laurie was the first person that showed genuine concern. She was very upfront with me and my financial situation, and the fact that I would not be able to attend that specific treatment center. But that is not where it ended. Laurie and I continued contact over the next several weeks, and she never gave up on me. One day I received an email from her about a treatment center in my area. I called immediately and made an appointment for my initial assessment. I was extremely excited when I realized this might actually work. Finally, a center that offered Intensive Outpatient Treatment at an affordable price. The next few weeks were extremely stressful. I wanted so badly to enter treatment, but still could not find the financial means to do so. Until I talked to my bishop at church. After many interviews, he determined this was something I definitely needed. Through the help of my church, a change in jobs, and the support of Laurie, I finally entered the treatment center.

Treatment was absolutely the hardest thing I have ever done in my life. I was blessed to work with the most amazing therapist I had ever met. Samantha** was genuinely concerned about me and my recovery. She never gave up on me, and always had more faith in me than I ever could have imagined having for myself. She pushed me to the limit, and then encouraged me take one more step. Samantha always knew I had it in myself to pull through this, and she was not going to allow me to lose sight of those possibilities. One day we decided it was time for me to give up the diet pills and laxatives once and for all. Both Samantha and I are very spiritual people, so we thought it would be fitting to have a "burning" during our spirituality class that week, and truly say goodbye to the poison. That is the one day in treatment that I will never forget. As I placed the pills into the bin, I was focused and determined to let that be the end of it. The fire was so symbolic, as I watched the smoke rise and the painful components floated away. I would like to share my journal entry from that day.

> I brought my diet pills and laxatives into treatment today. We all went outside, said a few words, and then I burned my stuff and everyone else wrote things on paper that wanted to get rid of and burned the papers as well. Then Samantha said some really nice things to us all and we had a moment of silence as we watched the smoke float away. I completely broke down! It was so crazy, the profound effect the burning had on me.

> When it was all over, Samantha came up and hugged me and told me that was the hard part and just to keep pushing thru the pain. I put my hands to my face because I was crying so hysterically, but Samantha took my hands, looked in my eyes and said I am doing an awesome job and to continue being strong. She hugged me again and whispered, "they're gone, Sarah. They're gone." All of a sudden, I was overwhelmed by a feeling of gratitude. Those 5 simple words were all I needed to hear, and the fear and anxiety just disappeared.

From that point on, I worked my hardest every day. I listened intently while in group and did my best when not at the center to keep myself on track. I continued having great days, days of complete breakthroughs and saying goodbye to Ed. One weekend my mom even came to the center with me for a day and we had a session with Samantha. It was absolutely amazing to have that time with my mom. To tell her how I truly felt, to have her understand what I was going through, and feel of her love and support. A few days later I had yet another breakthrough day at treatment. I can remember leaving that afternoon and having a completely over-whelming feeling of genuine happiness. I could not stop smiling and laughing! I still am not sure where this epiphany came from, but I will never forget that day. To my core I felt a complete sense of gratitude and happiness and insight into my new life without Ed. This is my journal entry from that amazing day.

> Having a pretty good week so far. Treatment has been really great; groups everyday that have been very insightful and educational. I have been doing really good with my eating and am feeling great emotionally as well. I am starting to feel normal again and am learning to identify my emotions again

and am realizing how much of a miracle my body and my life truly are. It's such an amazing feeling to see that my life, right now today, is very worth living. With every scar, every wound, every speed bump and bad day and ugly situation, I am becoming the person that God meant for me to be. I am finally able to embrace that fact and love that person!

I graduated from treatment 6 months ago after 8 weeks. I now have a new life. My life is so much more amazing, more poignant, amazing and beautiful without the negative effects of Ed. My body is a miracle, it is a gift, and I am finally learning to treat it with the same love and respect I would give to others. I realize my potential and know that I can not fulfill those goals without the miracle of my physical body. My skin is the home to my spirit and soul and those are things I have learned not to take for granted. Everyday is a new day. I still have struggles, but that is the beauty of life. I am now more grateful for those struggles because I have regained my insight and am learning new lessons everyday. Ed still attempts to speak to me on occasion, but that is a voice I am well aware of and will not allow to take me over again.

I will be forever indebted to those people that have helped me along the way. My parents have displayed unconditional love and helped me to see the truth. I never would have gotten this far without the help of amazing people along the way including, Jules***, Laurie and not to mention Samantha! Thank you for having the faith in me to push me to limits I never thought were possible. Our struggles in life are not meant to be faced alone. Thank you for never allowing me to feel alone, and never allowing me to give up on myself. My life is worth fighting for, and very worth living!

By Sarah Kipp, 26. Las Vegas, Nevada, USA. EDNOS (Eating Disorder Not Otherwise Specified) for 14 years. In Strong Recovery. If you want to get in touch with Sarah, feel free to send an e-mail to **slkipp@yahoo.com**.

---

* Laurie Daily is a certified eating disorder specialist and a professional singer. Some of Laurie's song lyrics are in this book.

** Name has been changed to protect person's privacy.

*** Jules is a friend of Sarah who is also recovering from an eating disorder.

My therapist gave me an assignment one week to write a letter to Ed, my eating disorder. Here is what I wrote:

Dear Ed,

I really wish you would get out of my life. I am fed up with your web of lies and deceit. You know, I do have to give you props because you are so good at what you do. How do you get to be such a good liar and fake? You must be really proud of yourself because I know you have worked your butt off to get to know every intimate part of me. Is it really that satisfying to know that the only thing you have accomplished in this life is destroying someone else's life?

You must be one jealous jerk, Ed, because if you look around yourself, you are among some of the strongest, smartest, and most accomplished people in this world. That's right, Ed, take a look around. Doesn't that make you feel small and ignorant?

I absolutely cannot believe that I fell for your game. You introduced yourself to me at the perfect time. In the middle of stress, anxiety, and my naïve quest for perfection, you stepped right in and picked up all the pieces. You think you are such a hero, don't you? What kind of hero can brainwash someone into believing that the skin I live in is the most important thing? What kind of hero can push someone to their absolute limit but still encourage them to accomplish the impossible? What kind of hero feeds a person complete, utter and ridiculous lies about being strong and independent?

You know what, Ed? You are the last person in the world that should be talking about strength and independence! Why? Because without me, you are NOTHING! Because without all of your innocent victims you would not have a leg to stand on. You thrive off of your games of degradation and deceit and trickery. You feed off the brilliant minds of beautiful people and lead them to believe that beauty is only skin deep.

Well, surprise, surprise Ed! I got your number and know your game. Wake up, Ed, because you no longer have me on cruise control. You will have to fight down to your last, dying breath to get hold of me again. And even then I will bite my way through your rope of lies and unrealistic expectations of me. I will no longer allow you to keep me in your death grip because I want to live!

I want to live free of the fear, anger, perfectionism and selfishness that you force on me. I want to love me; the complete me. The brilliant mind, the loving soul, the creative spirit that I have been blessed with. And most of all, I want to love the skin that all those powerful traits are housed in. I want to be strong both physically and emotionally. But I will never, ever be strong and independent as long as I allow you to creep in and corrupt me.

You, Ed, have accomplished absolutely nothing with me. Because in the end, when I am truly and completely through with you, I will be stronger, more confident and more beautiful than ever before. And I will do everything in my power to reveal the true Ed to the world and deny you any further opportunities to mess up someone else's life.

You are nothing but a cold, mean, timid little liar and the truth is that you will never measure up to the amazing lives you attempt to destroy. Good riddance, Ed. Move on because I am through with you. Look in the mirror, and remind yourself of who you really. Now I know the truth, I can see the truth and identify the reality of MY life. Because in the end, it is MY life and I will not associate with jerks who are out to mess me up and screw me over.

Sarah

By Sarah Kipp, 26. Las Vegas, Nevada, USA. EDNOS (Eating Disorder Not Otherwise Specified) for 14 years. In Strong Recovery. If you want to get in touch with Sarah, feel free to send an e-mail to **slkipp@yahoo.com**.

LETTING GO OF ED

The only way I've learned how to cope
Is through the eyes of Ed
Naively listened and fallen victim
To all the lies he said.
He grabbed on tight, held on for dear life
'Til I could no longer fight back
Led me down a dark road filled with only false hope
Showing me all the strength that I lacked.
But things are changing, the road dimly lit
I am finding myself through the haze
Building my strength and finding some hope
Looking forward to brighter days.
No longer obsessed with the weight of my skin
I'm finding the beauty and light deep within.
The fear that I feel no longer consumes
Each moment of each passing day
I have faith in myself, believe in myself
And my innate ability to change.
Each day gets brighter as each moment feels lighter
Renewing my hope and my faith
My life is worth living, my soul is worth saving
I will cherish each passing day.

By Sarah Kipp, 26. Las Vegas, Nevada, USA. EDNOS (Eating Disorder Not Otherwise Specified) for 14 years. In Strong Recovery. If you want to get in touch with Sarah, feel free to send an e-mail to **slkipp@yahoo.com**.

MESSAGE IN A BOTTLE

I stand naked and unafraid before you
I used to abhor you
Now I explore you
You show me the crinkle in my nose
You show me the belly that I hold
My head is up high, I am alive

I stand still and un-retouched
You loved me so much
I am enough
You were never the enemy
Just a reflection of my sanity

I've mistaken me in the past as an empty glass
Washed up on an empty sea, I tried to shatter you
But you always knew the truth
There's a message in the bottle

I stand naked and unafraid to touch you
I see right through you
There's so much inside you
You show me the softness of my skin
You show me it's just the flesh that I'm in

I've mistaken me in the past as an empty glass
Washed up on an empty sea, I tried to shatter you
But you always knew the truth
There's a message in the bottle

Oh, Lord, knows I've tried
To leave the image of time
You've implanted in my mind
Behind me
But instead, I've accepted what you said

By Laurie Daily. San Diego, California, USA. Recovered 14 years from all Eating Disorders. Laurie is a professional singer and Certified Eating Disorder Specialist who has dedicated her music to eating disorder recovery. All of the songs on Laurie's CDs relate to her own journey from eating disorders to heal in hopes to inspire others to live a life free from anorexia, bulimia, and compulsive eating. For more information, go to **www.lauriedaily.com** and **www.harmony-grove.com**. *"I've been there, I know how you feel. . . You can recover!"*

BEAUTY LIES WITHIN

What ya tryin to prove
Who you tryin to show
What you know
How far will you go
To be somebody
Everyday becomes a beginning
For you to compete
To feel complete
Ya gotta be better than
The day before
Ya gotta be more
It's all on the outside
You can hide
What you feel inside
But you gotta show them
You gotta blow them away
Someday
The way you look
The way you talk
The way you sing
The style you bring
What you do
Who you screw
You just knew
You gotta be the best
Better than the rest

Don't you know
It's just a show
And that I know, my friend
You gotta look inside
Stop running

Don't waste your time
Give up the fight
And you will find
That power you are seeking
Ah, Beauty Lies Within
Ah, Beauty Lies Within

So girl, you think you got the hair
The nails
But have you got the breasts?
Society will put you to the test
Are you toned yet you still feel alone
Silicone injected, infected,
& still neglected?
A little more a little less
Are you willing to confess
What you ingest
To keep the thighs
That go with that shape
Keepin your head in the toilet
Tryin not to spoil it
Cause you gotta compete to feel complete
And you look for the man
With the wallet in his hand
You screw and say "I do"
And you think you're safe
For a while
Doesn't matter that he cheats
Calls you a whore
& slaps you against the door
Cause his apology and all his theology
Dry your tears and make you smile
For awhile
Take a drink and something pink to help
You sink into sleep for awhile

Don't you know
It's just a show
And that I know, my friend
You gotta look inside
Stop running
Don't waste your time
Give up the fight
And you will find
The power you are seeking
Ah, Beauty Lies Within
Ah, Beauty Lies Within

Mr. Cool strives not only to be rich
But to chase that bitch everyone else is
Dreaming of
He's got the car, the cash, the vial
Full of hash
Or whatever love drug fashion bug that
The thug is into the day
He's got the toys, he hangs
With the boys,
Keeps up that macho superficial noise
But nobody knows what's inside
For he hides
Won't shed a tear
Never call him a queer
Take another drink, smoke,
Light up dope,
Try to make a joke
So no one will get under his masquerade
For he is alone
He is alone
Under all that muscle tone
But don't tell him he's got a problem
For he'll make you the blame,
Put you to shame,

Try to protect his name
But somewhere deep inside
He knows he can't hide

Don't you know
It's just a show
And that I know, my friend
You gotta look inside
Stop running
Don't waste your time
Give up the fight
And you will find
The power you are seeking
Ah, Beauty Lies Within
Ah, Beauty Lies Within

By Laurie Daily. San Diego, California, USA. Recovered 14 years from all Eating Disorders. Laurie is a professional singer and Certified Eating Disorder Specialist who has dedicated her music to eating disorder recovery. All of the songs on Laurie's CDs relate to her own journey from eating disorders to heal in hopes to inspire others to live a life free from anorexia, bulimia, and compulsive eating. For more information, go to **www.lauriedaily.com** and **www.harmony-grove.com**. *"I've been there, I know how you feel... You can recover!"*

WALK THROUGH THE RAIN

The storm is coming
And ya start to tremble
A dark cloud follows you
You tried to run before
You can't do that anymore
Teardrops start to fall
Can you handle it at all

The wicked wind
Rips through your heart
Emotions tear you apart
In the darkness there
When you feel like no one cares
Come take my hand
We'll lead you to dry land

Walk through the rain
When you got a friend
You can stand the pain
You'll be alright
You'll see the light
When you got a friend
You can walk through the rain

Thunder and lightning can't
Get to you
Got your brother and sister
Looking out for you
Through the darkest of storms
They will see through, so hold on
There is a rainbow for you

By Laurie Daily. San Diego, California, USA. Recovered 14 years from all Eating Disorders. Laurie is a professional singer and Certified Eating Disorder Specialist who has dedicated her music to eating disorder recovery. All of the songs on Laurie's CDs relate to her own journey from eating disorders to heal in hopes to inspire others to live a life free from anorexia, bulimia, and compulsive eating. For more information, go to **www.lauriedaily.com** and **www.harmony-grove.com**. *"I've been there, I know how you feel... You can recover!"*

The Secret I Was Not Allowed To Tell

By Nadia Lovell, 29. Wales, England. Anorexia and Bulimia for 12 years. Recovered. I have set up a self help group in Cardiff and am on the path of qualifying as a councillor so I am able to help others who are experiencing the distress of suffering from an eating disorder.

My recovery from an eating disorder took strength, patience, love, acceptance and courage; however I found all these qualities within my self. It is amazing of the inherent sense of survival that we all possess within us. In my deepest moments of despair when I just wanted to disappear, I never lost hope of the thought that one day I would find the key to the dungeon I was locked in for so many years. The dungeon of course being my mind, a mind consumed by obsessive eating, body loathing and self-hatred and this I did.

I made the choice to go beneath the symptoms of my eating disorder and to embrace the emotional wounds which I believe lie at the heart of all eating disorders. I learnt how to feel my emotions rather than mask them with overeating or under eating. I learnt to accept, love and care for my body rather than torture it for not conforming to the cultural expectation of being stick thin. I learnt the secret of loving myself despite having some fat on my belly.

When I made the choice to recover, I realised that I had a choice. Either I could continue on a cycle of self abuse with most of my days feeling numb, sad, lonely and isolated or I could take a leap into the unknown and discover what life had to offer without my obsession to be thin. I chose the latter because the pain of my eating disorder became too much, it wasn't working anymore. The euphoria I used to experience when losing a few pounds was slowly replaced with feelings of despair and hopelessness. I was ashamed of my inability to stop my eating behaviour but felt that I could not share my thoughts with anyone. I could not make any logic of my obsession; I already believed I was crazy. It was my secret, which I could not tell. However, I knew that the first step of recovery was to tell my story and when I made the commitment I felt that my prayers were answered as it was then I met my wonderful psychotherapist who literally held my hand as I ventured on my path of recovery.

My obsession with food began at the tender age of fourteen; it was my coping mechanism to deal with the difficult emotions that I was experiencing. I did not want to feel the anxiety and fear of beginning high school, of being accepted, making new friends, being successful academically. I did not know how to express my feelings; I came from a family like many others which was not comfortable in talking and dealing with emotions. But this attitude did little for my confidence as I became more insecure and was constantly plagued with thoughts of not being good enough. I believed that if I could change the contours of my body then everything about me and my world would be fine. All my fears and anxieties would be stripped away and I guess they were as I became locked in a world of calorie counting and exercise. The world I created was in my eyes safe, as long as I was thin I did not have to feel the pain of my first boyfriend ending our relationship, I did not have to worry about my exams, I did not have to panic about growing up. However as the years went by my coping mechanism was not as effective as it once was, food no longer protected me from all my negative emotions by making me numb. Instead I constantly felt sad, lonely, scared, and desperate I forgot that joy, happiness, laughter, and peace existed.

I felt ashamed at not being able to obtain perfection. I had a voice in my head, constantly telling me that I wasn't good enough, I did not deserve to be loved, I was useless, It was all my fault, I should look better, I was fat, ugly and disgusting, there was something wrong with me. The messages were constant and I believed them. I would look around me and find plenty of evidence to support my imperfection, my unlovable nature and my worthlessness. No matter how hard I tried, no matter how thin I got, I never felt good enough. I believed that I did not deserve to be living, I was a complete failure, my life was a shambles, I was a waste of space.

When I made the choice to recover, I was filled with anxiety. Not only did I believe that I would never get better but I also believed that I wasn't that ill, there was still a part of me that questioned whether I really did have an eating disorder. Despite vomiting after every meal for the past 11 years I still questioned whether Bulimia was really that serious. There was a part of me that wanted to keep hold of my familiar friend; I was scared of what it would be replaced with. Obsessing about food was all I knew, who was I if I wasn't counting calories? All my hobbies were designed to lose weight; my eating disorder was my identity. I was petrified that recovery meant getting fat, my biggest fear of all. I could not comprehend how I could possibly like myself if I put on weight if I hated myself when I was at my thinnest!

This is the place that I learnt to trust. This is the point that I chose to face the fear and do it anyway. I was no longer convinced that being thin would give me the self esteem which I yearned for. By letting go of my need to be thin I made room for the underlying feelings to emerge. I worked closely with my therapist as I expressed my feelings of despair and hopelessness caused by the voice in my head which was constantly telling me that I was a fat, useless, worthless pig. We examined where the messages came from, which included critical parents, friends, boyfriends and teachers. I wanted to be loved and accepted and approved for being me, not for my achievements and perfect behaviour. I feared rejection caused by not being good enough, I realised that my physical appearance became my avenue of acceptance. My fear of rejection manifested into a huge fear of being fat. My therapist reassured me that I was not using food because I was undisciplined and I was wrong but because it was the only way that I knew how to take care of myself and to stop the pain caused me by the constant negative messages being played like a broken record in my head.

Following many sessions with my therapist, I slowly began to make peace with my inner critic. I replaced thoughts of judgment and criticism with thoughts of compassion and forgiveness. I began to experiment with alternative ways to take care of myself. When I was feeling sad I learnt just to sit with my feelings and allow myself to cry trusting that the feelings would past just like clouds that pass by in the sky on a summer's day. When I needed love and reassurance I learnt how to express my needs to my friends and relatives. I learnt how to sooth myself by meditating and relaxing in a warm bubble bath. I learnt to be kind and patient with myself. I let go of good and bad food and learnt the art of intuitive eating by listening to my body. I ate when I was hungry and stopped when I was full and I also learnt to accept my body.

There were many times I felt that I was taking one step forward and ten steps back, but that is the road of recovery. It is tough but hugely rewarding at the same time. The key is to trust the process and to never stop believing that recovery from an eating disorder is possible. Eating disorders are not about food, that is why staying focused on the symptoms does not work. Anorexia, bulimia and overeating are coping mechanisms put in place to suffocate a desperate need for unconditional love, approval and acceptance by others and our selves. By choosing recovery, you take the risk of loving yourself from a deep sacred place within; very few people are given this chance. Many people live their lives, without questioning the meaning of self love and acceptance. They live a life of mediocrity, not really liking them selves but at the same time not particularly hating themselves. I hear of women all over the world constantly on a diet believing that when they loose the extra half a stone they will be happy. Your eating disorder is screaming at you to live an amazing life filled with love joy and compassion. The more of these qualities you possess in yourself the more love you attract into your life. But first you must make the choice either to stay locked in a prison of pain and torture masked by the numbness of over or under eating, or to take a leap of faith and feel the pain, sadness, hopelessness, self hate and desperation which is at the root of all addictions including eating disorders. I thank my eating disorder each day because I believe that without it I would not have questioned why I hated myself so much and without asking this question I would never have been thrown on the path of learning the secret of self love and when you possess this quality the world becomes a far more beautiful, wonderful and inspiring place to live.

By Nadia Lovell, 29. Wales, England. Anorexia and Bulimia for 12 years. Recovered. I have set up a self help group in Cardiff and am on the path of qualifying as a councillor so I am able to help others who are experiencing the distress of suffering from an eating disorder. If you want to get in touch with Nadia, feel free to send an e-mail to **nadialovell@yahoo.co.uk**.

I'M THE GIRL

I'm the girl
you'd think was perfect
would never mess up
have pain to hide.

I'm the girl
you thought would never hurt herself.

I'm the girl
crying inside
throwing up after meals
dying at times.

I'm the girl
who needs your help
a loving hand
a tender heart.

I'm the girl
hiding in the corner
cuz I am not who u think I am.

By Krystal Malisheske, 18. Sartell, Minnesota, United States. Bulimia and Anorexia for 2 years. Recovered.

Take Heart

By Angela C., 19. Pennsylvania, USA. Bulimia. Anxiety and Depression. In Strong Recovery.

The first time I was unsatisfied with my body, I was ten years old. I developed very early, and was fully developed by the time I hit fifth grade. Most girls I knew didn't even begin to hit puberty yet. That same year began the teasing and tormenting by my peers that didn't cease until I finished high school. They made fun of my breasts, insisting that I stuffed my bra. I received nicknames such as "stuffy" and "faker". As I result, I became a social outcast for most of my schooling and had few, if any, friends at any given time.

I became terribly depressed. School was miserable, and despite my wonderful family, home was miserable as well. Even though I come from a very loving home consisting of two married parents and an older sister, I made my home life miserable by frequently acting out and rebelling. How foolish we are when we are young. I now know how caring they are, and would never think to intentionally disrespect any of them. I was always into some kind of trouble, whether at school or at home. Detention was a frequent hang out, and my academics suffered severely. I also began to experiment with boys and my sexuality. Even though I never had sex until I was fully ready, I began to "push the limits" with many boys, most of whom I didn't know well.

Things became so bad that my family spent money out of pocket to seek help for me, even when no money was available. I needed psychiatric help because I was so suicidal. Fifth through eighth grade were the lowest years of my life, and I hope never to experience a fraction of the helplessness and despair of what I felt during that time.

My family had the sense to keep me involved in the church we attended, which had an active youth group. Many of the friends I met through the church are still some of my best friends today! The church environment planted the seeds that led me to keep a strong faith in God that sustains me today.

I still remembered the first time I vomited after eating. After youth group, our church hosts an all-church dinner. I sat and ate with my friends, many of whom were affluent and who always wore stylish clothes. At the time, materialism was quite important to me. I realize only now how silly it seems not to be comfortable in your own skin. I did not think I was attractive physically in any sense of the word and knew the only part of my outer appearance I could change was my body. I vomited in the church bathroom. I acted partially to lose weight, and partially out of utter despair. I had no other way of letting out my emotions.

My binging and purging episodes continued off and on from when I was 11 until I was 18. Sometimes, I vomited several times a day, whatever I ate. Sometimes, however, it was only weekly. Binging came whenever I was lonely, bored, or anxious. I ate thousands of calories mindlessly in one sitting. The funny thing is, I never realized I had a problem during this time. One thing that defined my personality during late high school was over-achieving. I kept a 4.0 GPA and was heavily involved in my community, and continued to serve in and through my church. I kept busy by staying in clubs and activities, even taking a leadership role in a few of them. I loved working to earn extra cash, so I was always employed. As a result, I won a plethora of scholarships which enabled me to go to college. By the closing of high school, I was in a right relationship with my family and God. I was getting along better with my parents who became less concerned, and more proud. I was also very thankful to graduate, which enabled me to escape the school life which had troubled me so much. Even in my latter teen years, though, food was problematic for me. I didn't like my appearance, and didn't quite know how to deal with it. As a bulimic, my body weight fluctuated within a normal weight. I always carried around a few more pounds than the rest of my friends. I didn't binge as often as I used to, but I definitely continued to purge.

I first knew that I had done some real damage to my body the summer after my senior year. I began getting frequent sore throats and had a general feeling of being run down. In addition, I missed my period twice in a row. I knew I wasn't pregnant because I never had sex. I skipped menstrual cycles because of my actions.

Then came college. College was a completely different scene than high school. I made many friends, succeeded in school, and fit right in. I was finally more at ease with myself. Even though college is notorious for stereotypically gorgeous girls, I was fine just being me. Though I had a few boyfriends in high school, I found my dream date in college. He was handsome, athletic, and extremely intelligent. In fact, we are still dating!

I went to college hoping to stop my behaviors. I had to. One functions best when one is healthy. It is incredibly difficult to break a habit of that nature, but I did it! I went a few days without purging, then I relapsed. Then a few weeks, then relapse. Then a few months, then relapse. Finally, with many prayers and a strong will to survive came victory. I've gone six full months without purging, and nearly two years without doing so on a regular basis.

College is a different environment than any other. All of the freedom of adulthood exists, but with few of the responsibilities. It is comparable to a "buffer zone" for the real world. It is incredibly easy to make poor decisions, but there's also a drive to better oneself. I chose the route to better myself. I am maintaining a 3.85 GPA with a 4.0 in my major. I work two jobs and am heavily involved on campus. I am even an RA! I get to mentor other girls!

Take heart: recovery is difficult, but it is certainly plausible. I overcame the depths of depression to enjoy some of the finest times of my life. I am having a blast with my new found self confidence. I have so many blessings all around me. I am still learning but coming closer to believing every day that it is truly what is on the inside that counts. After all, I look the same, but I have friends now because my outlook changed. Not everything is flowers and daisies, however. Sometimes I find myself down and occasionally questioning my appearance. Above all, I am happier now than I have ever been.

When you feel like no one cares, pray. When you feel like no one understands, pray. When you feel like you are at your rock bottom, pray. See a pattern? God will guide you to freedom much in the same way he's guided me.

By Angela C., 19. Pennsylvania, USA. Bulimia. Anxiety and Depression. In Strong Recovery.

YOU ARE PRECIOUS

You are loved far more than you know
So use your mind to learn and to grow
Feed your heart, your body, your soul
For you are the one that is in control
Today is the day that you must decide
Who you'll become and for what you will strive
You are so precious to God and to man
Someone will always be holding your hand
You are so beautiful, so sweet; yet so broken
Tears have shed; words have gone unspoken
Use your past for you, it is all you possess
Always look forward, don't you ever digress
Don't seek perfection, it'll steer you wrong
Seek out the challenges that make you strong
You are accepted, just as you are
Pray each night on each bright star
For forgiveness and faith, mercy and grace
God has created someone he could never replace

By Angela C., 19. Pennsylvania, USA. Bulimia. Anxiety and Depression. In Strong Recovery.

My Story

By Anita Humphries, 26, engaged. Birmingham, United Kingdom. Anorexia for 2 years and Bulimia for 8 years. Sexual Abuse. Self-Harm. Depression and Social Anxiety. Recovered.

My story begins very early in childhood in order to understand the vulnerability I felt from an early age. I was a middle child and always felt like I wasn't special. My parents never treated me badly but often I felt left out and isolated. My older sister had a lot more authority than me. She was allowed to try a lot of things and do a lot as she was the first born and the first to try everything.

My younger sister was the baby of the family. She was spoilt and got everything she wanted. I was the middle child for a long time and I had nothing to offer. I was often seen as the trouble maker and got blamed for most things. My sisters clicked onto this pretty quick and would often gang up on me and blame me for a lot of things (only silly childish things like drawing on the wall). As a young child I wasn't an angel but I was nowhere near as bad as I was made out to be.

I also felt the pressure on me was different to my sisters. My older sister was never really pressurised as she was effectively the guinea pig going through everything first. My younger sister was never expected to do anything as she was the baby or too young. However I felt I had a lot more pressure to succeed and also to help out in the house.

These early feelings I had set up for myself, only served as making me more vulnerable to the things life had to throw at me.

My first 'trauma' was when I was 9 years old. I went into a new class and had a new teacher. The teacher was a long-term supply teacher as the teacher who should have been teaching our class had left suddenly. From the very first day of meeting this teacher, she took an instant disliking to me and made sure I knew. I wasn't allowed to sit by anyone, as I was a "Distraction". I had to work and sit alone. If I tried to talk to anyone, I would get in trouble or chucked out of the classroom. I wasn't allowed to do the same work as the rest of the class. I had to copy poems from a thick poem book and they had to be perfect otherwise she would make me re-write the poems again and again telling me my writing was not good enough. On occasions she ripped up my work in front of the whole class telling me it was "rubbish" and "this is how not to do your work". She constantly told me I was stupid and that no one would want a child like me. She told me I was a trouble maker.

I told my parents about the teacher and they came up to the school. At first they were told I was making it up for attention, but eventually the head teacher agreed to observe one lesson. However he pre-warned the teacher about this and this was the only lesson she was ever nice to me. This meant I was branded a liar and the teacher's response to me was "no one will ever believe a stupid little child like you". She also told me she felt sorry for all the people who had to put up with me.

I had to put up with this for a year. I stopped attending school regularly for that year. On average I turned up about 2-3 days a week. I use to pretend I was ill but after a while I came to believe I was really ill. At this time, I also began to feel depressed and over the time it just continued to escalate. I remember feeling so depressed that I told my mum at 9 that I didn't want to grow up and I wanted to die. This was greeted with don't be so stupid or silly as they didn't know what else to say.

My parents kept taking me to the doctors as I was always telling them I was ill. I visited so often that my doctor told my parents I was a hypochondriac and that for a 9 year old to believe this, meant there were serious problems. This was ignored as I think they found it difficult to cope with.

This incident at school meant I lost all trust in adults but at this point I still trusted my peers. However this was soon to change when I started secondary school at age 11.

I was very different to my peers. I was quiet and withdrawn. My peers soon picked up on this and decided to let me know I was different. They bullied me.

At first the bullying was name calling. I was called a "freak" and "fatty". Though the name calling hurt I said nothing, just further re-drew into myself.

The name calling soon changed to physical violence. I was regularly beaten up. I was pushed, pulled, kicked and punched. I remember being tripped up and then being kicked while on the ground. I remember having my arm twisted so far up my back that it nearly broke.

As with most schools the teachers were aware that there was a bullying problem but the school's discipline was very poor and many teachers overlooked what they saw. I never said anything as I was scared. I just tried to hide and avoid them. This went on for four years of my secondary school life.

However the main bullying I will never forget is within that time. One lad decided to start sexually abusing me. I was 12 years old and it went on for 10 months. He touched me, fingered me and inserted various objects into me. He made me touch him as well. He hurt me both physically and mentally. I was left sore, bleeding and feeling dirty and used. I didn't say anything as I was scared of him. At first he told me if I said anything he would beat me up but I soon came to realise he was going to beat me up no matter what. I told him this and his response was that no one would ever believe me. He told me he would say I asked for it and consented and that's what people would believe. I believed him, so why wouldn't other people. He also told me no one would ever want me and this is the best I was ever going to get. He told me I was ugly, fat and a freak. The abuse stopped suddenly after 10 months and I never questioned why he stopped but was more grateful it had stopped.

Within this time I was also involved in a quite serious car crash. It was just before the abuse started. My dad was driving and the brakes failed. He lost control of the car and it turned over many times until eventually landing on its roof. My seat belt jammed and I was trapped inside and all I could hear was people shouting "quick get out, the petrol is leaking". I was petrified. I was lucky to get out with just shock but I wanted to talk about it but no one would listen. I still saw the images of being in the car turning around and around for a long time after this event.

By the time I was fourteen I felt terrible. I hated myself as I felt that I was to blame for everything that had happened. I was repulsed at who I was and wanted to change.

I believed that if I lost weight, as I was slightly overweight, that people would like me and I would start to feel different.

I started to diet and restricted my daily calorie intake. I also exercised excessively. I walked the long journey to school every morning, exercised in my room every night before bed and I spent my weekends swimming in the local pool.

The weight dropped off quickly. By the time I was 15, I was severely underweight. Looking back now I can see I looked terrible but at the time I couldn't see that. My rib cage stuck out, as did my hip bones. My eyes were sunken, my jaw bone had become very pronounced and my cheeks were drawn in. My hair was falling out and my nails had stopped growing. I was pale and weak, and often passed out. However I still saw this horrible fat, ugly thing and refused any help.

At the time, loads of people tried to tell me that I had a problem but I ignored any help. To me, I didn't have a problem and I thought people wanted to make me fat. People constantly went on at me and tried to make me eat. The constant threats I received about food meant I soon became scared that they were going to try and stop me. I needed to find a way to prevent this from happening, so I started eating in front of people who questioned me.

At the age of 16 I began eating more to satisfy people but nothing had changed inside. I needed to get rid off the food. This is when I started taking laxatives and I changed from Anorexia to Bulimia. I started of at taking small amounts of laxatives at first but this soon increased. A year into taking laxatives, I just craved food all the time. The meals I was eating were not enough to satisfy these cravings. It became impossible to satisfy my need for food, so I gave into it and had my first binge. Eating a large amount of food was great and ecstatic, it was like someone had given me a happy pill but this feeling did not last long. I felt bloated and disgusted with myself. I was repulsed with what I had just done and I needed to get rid of everything. For the first time ever at 17, I made myself sick and it felt great. From this point on there was no turning back. I stopped eating regular meals again and instead replaced each meal with a binge followed by purging.

I also found that the binging/purging helped me through coping with an attempted attack and mild racism. When I was 17, I was on my way to college when a strange man followed me and tried to attack me. I was lucky to come out with just a bruised a leg but it left me very shaken and no one would talk to me about it, just like no one would talk about the car crash. I needed to say what was on my mind.

Also the college I went to, was an inner city college and mainly full of Asian students. Black and white were in the minority. Being white I had never experienced racism before, so it was a bit of shock when people wouldn't talk to me at college due to my colour of my skin. However this didn't deeply affect me, as I managed to make friends and just ignored the racist people but it did mean that in my already vulnerable state I turned more to binging to make me feel better.

It was also at this time I stopped going out unless I had to. I avoided social situations and the thought of being in any social situation made me anxious causing me to have panic attacks. I was so concerned all the time about meeting people as I always thought they would be judgemental and criticise everything I do. I had developed social anxiety.

The binging/purging, to start with, felt wonderful and I was comfortable with what I was doing. I was controlling my weight but eating at the same time. I had put on weight due to eating again but I was still borderline underweight, which made me feel safe. The binging/purging was also a way to cope with everything that had happened and the feelings I had associated with this. However, by the time I was 19, the cycle of binging, purging and laxatives were starting to take its toll. I was spending most of my day binging and purging. I also spent most of my day on the toilet as I was taking excessively high amounts of laxatives daily. I was in a lot of pain, very tired and weak all the time. My moods were all over the place and I often found it very difficult to control them. I was also not going anywhere unless I really had too and when I did go anywhere I panicked at the slightest thing.

My moods had begun to affect me so much that I did not go straight to university and when I tried to do a course, I just found it too hard. I therefore decided not to continue with university and a week before my 20th birthday I got a job as a checkout supervisor. I thought getting this job would give me some control back into my life but this was not to be the case. A lot of people were not pleased I had got this job, especially three of my fellow supervisors who thought I was too young to be a supervisor and didn't like any of the ideas I put forward. They decided to make my time there as difficult as possible in the hope I would give up and leave. They would often make the work I had done disappear, so I would get in trouble. They also failed to tell me about any changes, so that again I would get in trouble by the managers. I hated the job but needed the money.

However, mentally inside I was at breaking point and on the 20th of June, 2000 I had had enough. I was severely depressed and seriously bulimic. I hated life and didn't want to live anymore. I took an overdose of painkillers and some more laxatives. I took the overdose when I should have been at work and went missing, which meant people were searching for me. I eventually went to hospital myself as I felt guilty that I would hurt my parents and agreed to treatment.

The overdose hit my family hard. My dad refused to see me at first and my mum couldn't stop crying. I started to regret the treatment. I wanted to be dead. Recovering after the overdose was one of the hardest things I have ever done. To still be here when you expect to be dead is hard to explain. Also, on that day everything but the sexual abuse came out. My parents couldn't cope and things were hard. It was soon after this I started to self-harm as I needed something to help me cope with all the pain and out of control feelings I was having.

I was referred to a psychiatrist and an eating disorder clinic in Birmingham but neither were any good. The eating disorder clinic just concentrated on my weight, not my feelings and the psychiatrists just wanted to give me sleeping pills, anti-depressants and any tablet to keep me dozy. I needed to change this and decided to return to education and go to university. I moved away against everyone's wishes but I needed to get out of that situation. That is when I came back to Bangor, North Wales (I had already started and given up a degree before in Bangor).

The help I received at Bangor was exceptional. I began seeing a doctor on a regular basis who managed to get me referred to a psychologist. However, the start of my recovery did not go well. When I first went into therapy at Bangor I had no intentions of recovering. I was only going along with therapy as it was a condition attached to my degree. I was studying to become a teacher and I had only been accepted on the basis I started therapy. Due to this attitude, things never really improved. I panicked at the slightest thing, I was often depressed to the point of being suicidal, my daily laxative intake was excessive, I spent all my spare time binging/purging or cutting and I never went out unless I had too. On top of all this, the sexual abuse I had suffered came out during therapy in March 2001, which made life harder. I was struggling to cope again and it had become obvious.

However, things soon started to change. In October 2001 I met someone, who I am now engaged to. He was caring and understanding. He didn't run away when he found out about all my problems and seem to genuinely like me for who I was. This was the first positive thing I had felt in a long time and brought me back of the brink of suicide. I still struggled on though and in February 2002 I was declared mentally unfit to teach and was told to leave my university course for a break. Now at this point things could have gone either way as my depression hit rock bottom. However, with the support of my boyfriend, now my fiancé, I got through this and started to make the first positive steps to my recovery. I started to take therapy seriously as something to help me and I opened up more. I decided I would return to university to get a degree but I would change courses and wait until September 2002. This meant I could then concentrate fully on my recovery.

I started to cut down on my binging/purging and made attempts at stopping to self-harm. I started taking medication properly for my depression and anxiety (I had been given medication before but often missed doses or threw them away). As well as receiving individual therapy and support from my doctor, I also did a six month group therapy course. All of this helped me to stop binging, purging and self-harming though it did take time and there were many difficult moments throughout. It also helped me control my moods. However, I was reluctant to stop the laxatives as this was the only control I felt I had. I didn't know what I would be without them and it scared me to think of life without them. The final push I needed to seriously look at my laxatives was when my doctor told me would be dead by the time I was 25 as my body was not replacing the water quick enough that the laxatives were taking away. I was only 23 and it made me think seriously for the first time – did I really want to die after coming so far and meeting some-one I had grown to love? The answer to this was no, so I then started to gradually reduce the number of laxatives I was taking. I had to do it gradually both for my mental sanity but also physically. The number of laxatives I was taking meant that if I just stopped my bowel would have failed and water would have built up internally, potentially meaning serious illness if not death.

By my 24th birthday in January 2004 I stopped taking all laxatives and by March 2004 I finished the therapy I had started in 2001 and stopped taking my medication. I also finally completed my degree in June 2004, gaining a high pass with honours (without recovery I probably would have never got this).

It has now been two years I have been recovered and the feeling is great. I have more time as I'm not spending time cutting, binging, purging and sitting on the toilet. Though my moods are still all over the place they are easier to deal with and I'm now coming to terms with social situations, meaning I very rarely panic at the thought of one. I would be lying if I said recovery is easy and it has been plain sailing as it is the hardest thing I have ever done in my whole life. There have been moments in the last two years that I have slipped up and I have binged, purged, cut or taken laxatives but the difference now is these are one off events that I automatically deal with and prevent from happening again. It has taken me two years of being recovered to actually start to like myself and the way I look. To be honest I think I would love to lose some weight but I'm not letting that control me anymore. I have accepted that this is the way I look now. I am no supermodel and could never be one but who is to say that this image is correct. However, I know I am not fat and in the world of realistic women (i.e., not celebrities or supermodels), I am slim. Recovery is hard work but well worth every moment including the difficult parts.

By Anita Humphries, 26, engaged. Birmingham, United Kingdom. Anorexia for 2 years and Bulimia for 8 years. Sexual Abuse. Self-Harm. Depression and Social Anxiety. Recovered.

NO MORE
– AN AFFIRMATION OF LIFE

No more drama.
No more trauma.
No more victims.
No more hiding.
No more lying.
No more insanity ruling my mind.

No more self-sabotage.
No more denial.
No more guilt.
No shame.
No trying to gain unobtainable love.

No more conforming to be accepted.
No more bruises or black eyes.
No more being stranded barefoot in the rain in no-where-land.

No more ignoring my feelings.
No more ignoring my responsibilities.
No more being an emotional doormat.
No more looking back.
No more jails, hospitals, or rehabs.

No more cuts, burns or self-starvation.
A vow of life,
This I take!
No more pretending I don't matter.
No more reaching beyond myself to reach my dreams.
No more fooling myself that you're more important than me.

No more!

By Mara McWilliams, 37. Married with a ten year old daughter. California, United States. In recovery with a diagnosis of Bipolar Disorder, Panic Disorder, and Anorexia. Mara is an artist and expresses herself through painting and poetry. The freedom and release she finds in painting has been nearly as beneficial to her recovery as therapy. Mara's ultimate goal is to educate our society that through proper diagnosis, treatment, therapy, love, support, and understanding, recovery is possible. Please remember, as with any other illness, educating ourselves about our disorder is extremely important. For more information, go to **www. recoverythroughart.com.**

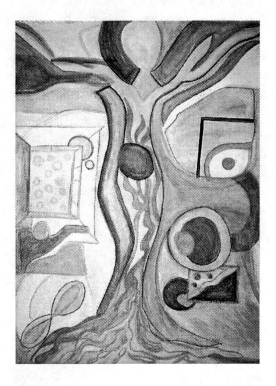

"Complete Woman" by Mara McWilliams, 37. Married with a ten year old daughter. California, United States. In recovery with a diagnosis of Bipolar Disorder, Panic Disorder, and Anorexia. Mara is an artist and expresses herself through painting and poetry. The freedom and release she finds in painting has been nearly as beneficial to her recovery as therapy. Mara's ultimate goal is to educate our society that through proper diagnosis, treatment, therapy, love, support, and understanding, recovery is possible. Please remember, as with any other illness, educating ourselves about our disorder is extremely important. For more information, go to **www.recoverythroughart.com.**.

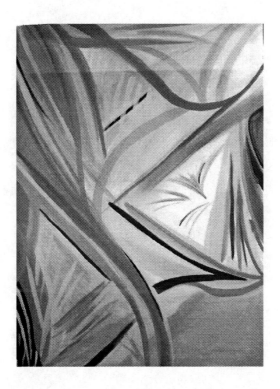

"**Recovery**" by Mara McWilliams, 37. Married with a ten year old daughter. California, United States. In recovery with a diagnosis of Bipolar Disorder, Panic Disorder, and Anorexia. Mara is an artist and expresses herself through painting and poetry. The freedom and release she finds in painting has been nearly as beneficial to her recovery as therapy. Mara's ultimate goal is to educate our society that through proper diagnosis, treatment, therapy, love, support, and understanding, recovery is possible. Please remember, as with any other illness, educating ourselves about our disorder is extremely important. For more information, go to **www.recoverythroughart.com**.

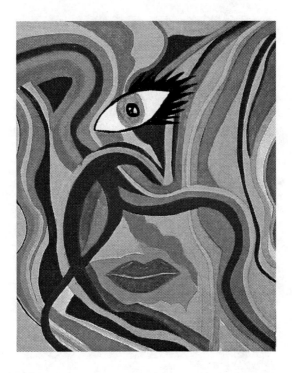

"Be One With All" by Mara McWilliams, 37. Married with a ten year old daughter. California, United States. In recovery with a diagnosis of Bipolar Disorder, Panic Disorder, and Anorexia. Mara is an artist and expresses herself through painting and poetry. The freedom and release she finds in painting has been nearly as beneficial to her recovery as therapy. Mara's ultimate goal is to educate our society that through proper diagnosis, treatment, therapy, love, support, and understanding, recovery is possible. Please remember, as with any other illness, educating ourselves about our disorder is extremely important. For more information, go to **www.recoverythroughart.com**.

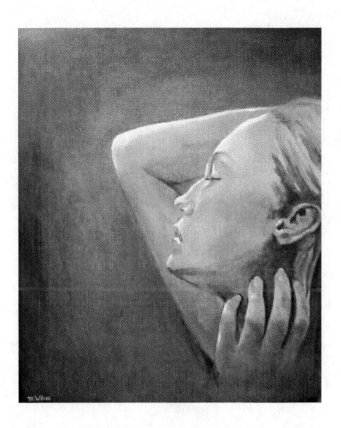

'**Reflection**' (Self-Portrait) by Michelle R Wilson, 28, Single. Vancouver, British Columbia, Canada. Anorexia-Bulimia for 10 years. Recovered however still occasionally challenged. Also history of Depression and Social Anxiety. Visual artist, focus on painting people. Currently work with adults with disabilities.

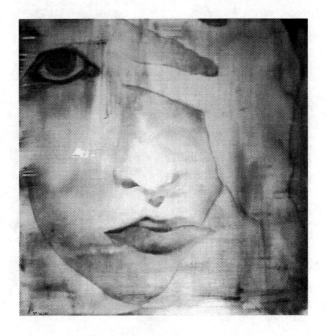

'**Searching**' by Michelle R Wilson, 28, Single. Vancouver, British Columbia, Canada. Anorexia-Bulimia for 10 years. Recovered however still occasionally challenged. Also history of Depression and Social Anxiety. Visual artist, focus on painting people. Currently work with adults with disabilities.

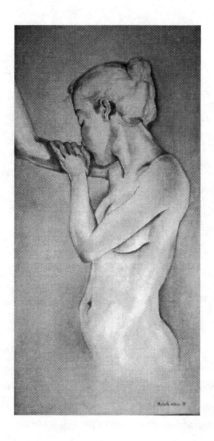

'**Healing**' by Michelle R Wilson, 28, Single. Vancouver, British Columbia, Canada. Anorexia-Bulimia for 10 years. Recovered however still occasionally challenged. Also history of Depression and Social Anxiety. Visual artist, focus on painting people. Currently work with adults with disabilities.

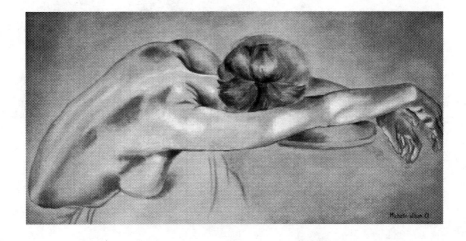

'**Resting**' by Michelle R Wilson, 28, Single. Vancouver, British Columbia, Canada. Anorexia-Bulimia for 10 years. Recovered however still occasionally challenged. Also history of Depression and Social Anxiety. Visual artist, focus on painting people. Currently work with adults with disabilities.

Please Don't Count Food Points in Front of the Children

By LA Crompton, 37, married, two children. New York, USA. Anorexia/Bulimia 10 years. Recovered 12 years.

It occurred to me this morning while absentmindedly eating a discarded bowl of Winnie-the Pooh cereal with a child-sized purple plastic spoon, that my eating habits have changed somewhat since becoming a mother. The realization sent me to the cupboard in search of a more respectable breakfast: my own bowl of Pooh cereal with an adult-sized metal teaspoon. While my tastes occasionally run toward the juvenile, I am grateful that deciding what to eat is no longer the super-charged emotional event it once was.

Adolescence marked my initiation into the prison of an eating disorder that morphed into every imaginable form over nearly ten years. I engaged in a war against my body because it began to grow more curves than I deemed attractive. In fact, judging by the fashion magazines I so cherished, my body was growing more curves than the world deemed attractive. And since my adolescent mind could not possibly realize that the world was wrong, and that my body was fine, I began a diet.

Diets teach us to mistrust the natural cues of hunger and fullness that our bodies send us. When diets are unsuccessful (which is nearly all of the time) they leave one feeling like a weak failure. We think there must be something wrong with us that we can't stick to a simple diet (no matter how ridiculous said diet may be). When diets are successful, they can sometimes become dangerous. The overwhelming approval one gets for losing weight can be unbelievably powerful. It can send one chasing after ever smaller numbers on the scale until one arrives at a weight far below the one God intended. This is what happened to me.

For a long time my life was reduced to a tunnel vision focus on what I ate. Even as I moved out of the all-consuming obsession of anorexia, I continued to perceive my body as disgusting and needy, all because it wanted to be fed. I hated it and saw it as my greatest enemy. I constantly tried diet after diet, looking for peace but was either cranky because I was hungry, or else cranky because I felt like a loser for eating. I could not become totally free until I began to question the infallibility of the skinny ideal.

I am grateful that the Lord granted me the wisdom to see my natural curves as beautiful long before I became a mother. It is, in fact, a miracle that after years of hating and starving my body it helped to bless me with a perfect little girl. When she was born and I felt that overwhelming love for her sweet precious body, I wept with the knowledge that the Lord looks at me with that same adoration. Looks at my body with the acceptance and love it once so craved.

If God intended mothers to have flat tummies, we would gestate our babies in our backpacks. And if we weren't supposed to have hips, we would carry our children around in pouches, not on the convenient hip-seats the Lord lovingly provides. Mommies are more fun to climb on when they are nice and soft, not all pointy and skinny. Thinking we cannot possibly love or accept our wonderful life-giving bodies until we lose ten or fifty pounds is truly 'following the hollow philosophies of this world.'

Seeing my little girl playing now so innocently, I cannot imagine her ever criticizing her sweet body. I look at the media and at the statistics and I know that the odds are very high that she will. (42% of first through third grade girls want to be thinner and 81% of 10-year-old girls are afraid of being fat.) My daughter very well may look down at that miracle of her body one day and see it through the world's eyes - as wrong. If she is built like her mother, she may be horrified by thighs too large and a butt too big - flaws as dictated by the mythological 'ideal.' Perhaps she will decide to try to change what she sees. Perhaps she will decide to hate what she sees. And I scream inside at the thought and want to claw down that wall the world builds between women and their own bodies. I want better odds for my daughter; I want her to see her body through my eyes as precious. To see it through the Lord's eyes as beautiful.

Imagine the pain of having your daughter tell you she doesn't like her body. The body formed in your womb that you prayed over and loved before she was born. Now imagine you are that daughter going to God, complaining about this lump or that curve and see His response. Take a minute out and thank your good body for serving you so well. Let your daughters see you loving and accepting your body AS IS, and perhaps they will have a shot at making peace with the women's bodies they will one day possess.

I have worked hard to appreciate my body and feed it freely. It has repaid me by finding a healthy natural weight that may not get me on the cover of any fashion magazines, but that enables me to keep up with an energetic toddler. I tune into what my body needs and oftentimes am surprised that it knows what to ask for: A huge variety of wholesome foods and sometimes Pooh cereal, all in balance, all taken in with love. Of the hundreds of messages received DAILY telling you that you need to change in order to be beautiful, I want to be part of the voice shouting above the din, "You are beautiful, just as you are!"

Just ask the Lord.

Just ask your kids.

By LA Crompton, 37, married, two children. New York, USA. Anorexia/Bulimia 10 years. Recovered 12 years. For more information, go to **www.dreamer-girl.com**.

GREEN EYES

I am admiring
a beautiful friend
whose coloring and build
are my polar-opposite
I am feeling
so plain and drab in her presence
I am sinking and hating
Until I am hit by the revolutionary
truth
that we can both be beautiful
Suddenly the lights go on
there is no such thing as fairest of all
we do not diminish each other
Jealousy is stupid
and pointless
and makes our brows furrow in a most
unattractive way
When I catch myself being jealous
or worse
trying to make someone jealous of me
I remind myself that jealousy
makes for cheap currency
and only the small-minded
use it for trade

By LA Crompton, 37, married, two children. New York, USA. Anorexia/Bulimia 10 years. Recovered 12 years. For more information, go to **www.dreamer-girl.com**.

GARDEN PARTY

The desert
is cheesecake
How could anyone loathe cheesecake?
Yet the women feign disgust
looking stricken
horrified by even the sight
holding up stop sign hands
in protest
shaking their heads
No, no, a thousand times
NO
As if the pale wedges could bite

Conversation turns
discussing flaws
comparing diets
Moaning
Whining
Must
Lose
Weight

I firmly tell these women
my sisters whom I love
that they are beautiful
Encourage them to recognize their beauty
To get on with their lives
forget about those
stinking
ten
pounds
While I slowly enjoy
a nice creamy slice
of cheesecake

By LA Crompton, 37, married, two children. New York, USA. Anorexia/Bulimia 10 years. Recovered 12 years. For more information, go to **www.dreamer-girl.com**.

One Girls Dream to Fit In

By Lisa Horsfield, 32. New Zealand. Bulimia for 10 years. In Recovery for 9 years.

I can still remember vividly the first time that I ever heard of anyone vomiting after they ate. I remember as a chubby 14 year old watching 'Different Strokes' where the teenage girl got caught vomiting after her meal and it went on to explain how dangerous it was to lose weight like this. I can remember thinking that night as I went to sleep and I prayed to god to please make me skinny and pretty as I did every night, but this night I remember thinking I wish I could learn to vomit, it would solve all my problems. Well let me tell you, solving problems it did not but it created a terrible, dark nightmare that was the result of one girls dream to fit in.

So began my journey of eating and then secretly going to the toilet and getting rid of everything. It wasn't so hard after a few failed attempts but I soon learnt the tricks. How to vomit quietly so as to let no one hear, what food came up the easiest and how to cover my tracks. What started off as an occasional purging soon evolved into a cycle of full on binging then purging episodes. When I looked in the mirror I saw a fat kid with long hair and big glasses and that's what everyone else saw too. I looked like the typical geek and I was reminded everyday at school. Kids can be so cruel; they really can make or break a soul. I used to stay in one spot over lunch so that people wouldn't see me. I had a big group of friends who accepted me but I always felt ugly. I can remember I was sitting on the school bus with my best friend and I just started crying. I told her what I had been doing and when I got to school I went to see the school councillor. Next moment I knew my mother and father were there and we were on our way to see a psychologist. Wow what a pile of crap that was, all they did was lay blame and all they were interested in was finding out why I was bulimic? I told them I did not know, 'it must be your parents, you must have some deep dark secret?', but I didn't. I didn't have the answers and all this blame just made me feel more guilty and more of a let down. My parents were wonderful people and I was brought up in a loving healthy environment and there was no one to blame. I had become a victim of society full of high expectations and peer pressure. I was a normal kid who had her own ideal of what was popular and acceptable.

So life just continued in a down hill spiral and by now I was starting to withdraw from my friends. I was skipping school, spending hours of my day binging and now I look back I feel I had lost my whole youth, what a waste, the best years of my life with my head in the toilet.

When I left school I moved to Australia and met my first boyfriend I was so in love, by now I was thin and had grown out of the gorky stage and here was a man who loved me for who I was, although he did not know my secret.

About two months after we started going out I decided to tell him, needless to say it did not go down well. "You should have told me before we started going out!" this insinuated that had I told him, he would not have been interested I was sure it was all over but we worked on it and although I don't think he ever truly understood or accepted my bulimia we learnt to live with it for a while. It did not help that he and his family had their own problems with alcohol so this was not the most productive environment and so although I knew my bulimia could make or break the relationship, I continued to spiral out of control to the extent where his mother rang the New Zealand embassy in Australia to ask them to help me. They said that as I was not an Australian citizen there was nothing they could do so I arranged to go back home to New Zealand on the advice of my boyfriend when he could no longer cope.

I was under the impression that I would be admitted into hospital but when I got home I was told that all that was available was a one hour counciling session once a week, two hours drive away. I remember being told that if it helped to take my mind off food that I should try masturbating which for an 18 year old was the most unexpected solution. He also told me to carry an apple to prevent me getting hungry, like hunger has anything to do with eating disorders! I was desperate and lonely and I missed my boyfriend. I felt like no one could or would help me so one night in share desperation I swallowed my bottle of antidepressants. I ended up in hospital having my stomach pumped but still there was no help. Here I was an 18 year old who had tried to kill herself and the very next day I was sent home! What has a girl to do around here to get some help? "HELP ME, DON'T YOU GET IT!?" So I continued to see the psychologist and although I stopped binging I continued to purge on a regular basis but it was enough to convince my parents to allow me to move back to Australia to be with my boyfriend. This as you could imagine was a disaster! I was back to square one within a couple of days, so after a couple of months I decided to move back home and although this took all my strength and caused a lot of pain I knew within myself, it was what I had to do for my survival. So I left my life in Australia behind me and although I was devastated to leave my boyfriend I know now that it helped save my life. I can remember my sister saying to me how strong I was to leave and give up the person I loved and even through all the pain, loved me back, but I had to, I had to protect my sanity as well as let him have the future he deserved with someone healthy without all the hang-ups that accompany this sad, cruel illness.

Three months after moving home on the day we buried my cousin having died from heart failure following years fighting anorexia I met the man who would nine months later become my husband.

I was very young, 19 years old but the bulimia still had its hold. He was very supportive, he never judged me, and he said I had an illness like anything else and we worked hard to overcome this demon but nothing seemed to work. No amount of therapy seemed to help but as time went on I started to realise that the issues of old had started to fad and now my condition was more of a habit than a psychological condition. When I was 23 my world changed forever I found out I was pregnant. How could I kill this thing living inside of me, this is my baby, part of me. How selfish can a person get putting her own needs, her own distorted views about herself in front of the life of her own baby? So this was the turning point in my life, this was my focus my reason to get better to not only save my baby but also myself.

So I stopped, don't ask me how but I could not bring myself to vomit and risk my baby. I went from vomiting a couple of times a day to virtually nothing, this baby was my saviour! So nine months later I gave birth to a healthy baby boy who is the joy of my life.

Many things have changed in the nine years that I have been in recovery and I say in recovery because I believe I will never be cured, it is always there in the back of my mind, I still watch what I eat and I am still finicky at times about food but it is controlled now.

My life is fantastic, unfortunately my marriage did not last but I believe I was too young and when I met my husband I was very quiet and as I got better I evolved, I grew up and I became a strong independent woman. I am now in the most wonderful relationship with a man who I adore and who I think the world of. My lovely, beautiful son now lives with his father although only 5 minutes away and I get to see him every second weekend and in the holidays. Oh how time flies, he is now nine and the most delightful child with whom I am most proud of. The son who saved me will grow up to be the man who has dreams and ambitions and who will always be the apple of his mother's eye.

I too had ambitions, I recently graduated and obtained a degree and I am now working as a registered nurse in a private hospital as a theatre nurse. I have come a long way from the deep dark centre of hell but I have made it. I am now a mother, a partner and a friend to many people and I am proud of who I have become and would not change any part of my life as I believe that all the things that are thrown at you, no matter how bad they are, are the very things that shape a persons integrity, their soul and their very being. So I can look at living through bulimia as a nightmare or I can look at who I have become and be proud of my life.

My name is Lisa Horsfield and I come from a little country called New Zealand and for 10 years of my 32 on this earth I suffered from bulimia but now I have been in recovery for 9 years and I wish all that read my story the best of luck and strength and guidance and I believe you will make it as I have.

By Lisa Horsfield, 32. New Zealand. Bulimia for 10 years. In Recovery for 9 years.

I Didn't Find What I Was Looking For In Hollywood, Paris or Milan...

By N.C., 30. Canada. Disordered Eating for 6 years. In Recovery. Practicing Mindfulness Mediation Daily.

My story starts at a later age than many people who suffer from a dysfunctional relationship with food. I am now able to see clearly that the seeds of my problem began as a small child, but the eating disorder itself first started making itself known in the summer after I graduated from university and started working as a catalogue and commercial model. I was twenty-four years old. It is now almost 6 years later and I can finally say that after a lot of hard work, spiritual reflection and faith, journaling, talking, listening, meditation, 'heart-to-hearts' with family, and self-reflection, I am making great progress in my recovery.

The story of my eating disorder begins in the summer of 2000. By 2003 it was an all-encompassing obsession. In 2004 I let go of all food restrictions and travelled a bumpy, binge-filled path to recovery. Since I was such a 'type A' person, I had actually given myself a "two year deadline" to recover from my eating disorder. I now realize that patience is one of the most important keys to full recovery. By 2006, I had finally figured out what was underneath it all and I can clearly see that I am developing a more and more balanced and grounded relationship with food as time goes by.

I still have my days where I indulge more than other days, and sometimes I still eat based on emotions rather than hunger, but I have realized that recovery is not a perfectly black-and-white, cut-and-dry thing. I don't believe that I will one day wake up to some glowing revelation that will make me never emotionally eat again from that point forward. But based on my experiences in recovery so far, and on talking to others who have recovered, I really believe that over these next couple of years I will continue to develop a more and more 'normal' relationship with food and when I have the occasional urge to indulge in a treat, I will feel less emotional about it. I am working on finding a comfortable spot somewhere in 'the grey area' of intuitive eating: not an all-or-nothing "overeater" or "perfect eater". I believe that I will continue along the path of strong and steady progress that I have been building on in the two and a half years it has been since I first walked into the Eating Disorder Information Center and began my recovery.

I had always been thin my whole life, sometimes awkwardly so. In my early twenties when a modeling agent first told me I needed to lose weight, I was a little surprised because I was already quite slim. How many times in later years would I wish I had never started my first diet.

I moved to Los Angeles in my early twenties to pursue a career in commercial modeling, and the glamorous life I thought would make me happy. My first year of working in modeling and TV commercials, I lost quite a bit of weight through minor dieting. It wasn't very hard for me because I had never really needed to diet before, so I didn't seem to feel deprived at that time. In my mind, it seemed like as I lost weight, doors were opening up for me and I found myself getting invited to lots of Hollywood parties and getting backstage at concerts and events. I later realized that none of those 'doors that were opening' were leading me anywhere closer to my goal of happiness, but that took quite a while to figure out.

One of my first and most memorable binges after I'd begun modeling, really took me by surprise. I was at a Hollywood Hills party of some wealthy young model I had met at a casting call and I was meeting all these well-known TV actors and people I felt kind of intimidated by. All of a sudden I found myself in her gourmet pantry, chowing down on food I hadn't been offered to eat. This wasn't me: I was the girl who didn't ever worry or care about food, who actually sometimes "forgot to eat" until my hunger would remind me I needed some food. What was I doing!?

I had also developed the habit of visiting the bakery to eat 2 or 3 "treats" after an audition or casting. Then I would reprimand myself and re-commit to exercising religiously and restricting my food more.

Later that year, when I travelled to Europe to try my luck in modeling over there, suddenly I found myself having uncontrollable urges to eat the "forbidden foods" I had been trying to stay away from for several months. The more I tried to stop myself and promised myself in the mirror that I would be stricter, the more I felt compelled to eat. My idea at the time was to counterbalance this with exercise, and I often found myself either jogging or at the 24-hour gym into the wee hours of the night. I had no idea what was going on with me and all I knew was that this cycle was started to make me feel unbalanced. But would I ever imagine I had a problem with my eating behaviors? No way!

In Europe, many of the models I met seemed to be feeling as bad, or worse than I was. There may be many grounded, happy and successful models out there who are strong and balanced enough to make it work in the industry. They say "birds of a feather flock together" and I was probably attracting all the models who were going through as hard a time as I was, so my story is by no means representative of a typical model, especially since I only worked in the industry for about one and a half years and I had my own self-esteem challenges long before starting the job.

One of my friends had the daily habit of snorting some kind of drug she had brought over with her to Paris. She told me one of the biggest challenges in her modeling lifestyle was acting "normal" at casting calls or when meeting with agents, when she was high. Her drug supply ran out and she was devastated to put on an incredible amount of weight in a short period of time. Another model I hung out with who was doing runway work for a very famous lingerie company, was a self-professed "former heroin junkie". Other girls talked about models that were young, suicidal, confused and so homesick. One girl told me about her "stunning and successful" model friend who had killed herself after being used by men and giving up hope.

Some typical conversations I would hear around the hotel where the models stayed were: "Do you know how to lose weight fast? My agent wants me to lose XXX pounds by next week. How much do you weigh? I came here for a month to lose weight before I head back to Paris. What did you eat today? I can't go for a walk with you because I don't want my legs to get muscular before the spring fashion shows. And on and on....."

My last month of modeling in Europe was particularly disturbing. I started hanging out with a very wealthy, probably mafia-connected older man who let all the models eat and drink all the alcohol they wanted in his restaurant for free every night. He also had a seemingly endless supply of cocaine and I am the kind of person who has a tendency to binge on things that let me avoid my feelings. I had some scary experiences when this guy decided that he wanted to pursue me, and this led me on my first long-term food "bender", which was a few weeks long!

By the end of the year, I returned home, feeling emotionally exhausted, defeated, and weighing more than I ever had before. My binge-drinking, eating and drugging was at an all-time high. Although I was trying to use these habits to help me not have to endure upsetting feelings, it was clear to me that I was completely messed up. But, within a few short months of being back home and nurtured by my boyfriend and friends, and because I was so dead-set on being thin, somehow I found myself losing the weight again and getting more modeling work than I had before.

After being knee-deep in the modeling industry and the L.A./Europe 'A-List' Party scene for a year, I was thoroughly convinced that the fast track to happiness and lifelong satisfaction rested with my ability to be as thin and pretty as possible for as many years as I could, and after that I would be ready to die. I never even considered things like the repercussions of the various ways I was abusing my body: chaotic eating, 'recreational' substance abuse, tanning salon overuse, overexercising with food still undigested in my stomach, brief experiments with diet pills. I refused to consider the fact that I would one day be dealing with the consequences of this abuse. My attitude was "I don't want to hear about it. I don't care. I just want to look good and live life to the fullest while I'm young. I'll worry about all that other stuff if and when I ever get to be old. "

When I booked my first catalogue lingerie photo shoot, I felt kind of guilty knowing that I had to "extreme diet" for 3 days before the photo shoot in order for my body to look the way it did in those pictures. It was around then that I realized that I was 'part of the problem' of young girls having unrealistic expectations for how they should look, based on what they saw in print ads.

By this time I was well into what would become my eating disorder pattern: binge on chocolate, cookies, ice cream or whatever each day, and then exercise compulsively for at least a couple of hours every day to try to burn off the calories. Because I had a naturally fast metabolism, and possibly because I was sometimes using drugs and alcohol as my "binge of choice", I was able to pull this habit off to some sad extent, for a couple of years and maintain a very fragile shell of "normalcy" around me. (Or so I thought.) But my brain was becoming an increasingly polluted and miserable place. Although I was having somewhat controlled "mini-binges" every single day, it was never even close to enough to satisfy me. I often thought to myself "how many chocolate bars and cookies would it really take to satisfy me if I didn't control myself?" The thought scared me.

I went back to Europe to try to get more modeling work and ended up hooking up with a male model who told me about a certain drug he was using to stay lean. I tried that drug, but it never did work for me. I decided to stick with my compulsive exercising. Then I started dating a wealthy businessman and I thought I had everything I had ever dreamed of: a billionaire boyfriend, VIP access to most events, a great wardrobe full of 4 inch designer stilettos (very comfortable), a thin body, a (not particularly successful) career in modeling, and a glamorous lifestyle. But there were just a couple of problems: I didn't really like my boyfriend, I had a compulsive eating disorder and I couldn't stand myself.

It was the summer of 2001. A good friend of mine gave me a book to read about meditation and the spiritual path. I couldn't believe it when everything the book talked about described exactly what was missing in my life. Reading that book set in motion somewhat of an identity crisis and opened my mind to a whole new outlook on life which was irreversible. Although I felt somewhat spiritually inspired, I did not feel at all comfortable with the idea of changing my lifestyle. I got fired from a job that autumn, and that set me off on another long-term binge-ing bender. I decided that the answer to my problems was liposuction, so I set up an appointment to get the surgery on my tummy, upper arms and under my chin, although my surgeon advised me that I didn't really need it.

I decided to return to L.A. for some more club-hopping and entertainment in-dustry excitement. By this time my modeling career was floundering, so I started working as the personal assistant to a big Hollywood manager.

I decided to become increasingly restrictive with what I ate. First I went vegetarian, then I became a "whole-foods-only, no sugar vegetarian", then I be-came a "raw-food vegan" then I started compulsively doing long-term juice fasts. Towards the end of this phase, I started doing long water fasts, where I had no en-ergy to do anything besides sit around all day. In between these extremely restric-tive phases, I would, of course, be binging on anything in sight. I read somewhere that "every diet has an equal and opposite binge", and I proved that to myself time and time again, but I still didn't get it.

I went to see a couple of hypnotherapists with the goal of making myself magically have no more urges to binge. It didn't work at all. I even called my two closest friends and made a solemn vow on our friendship that I would never binge again; that didn't work either. I did not have any tools to change my life and I was hoping for some kind of divine miracle to make it all go away, still in total denial that I could possibly have an eating disorder.

I started becoming really aware that it was impossible for me to enjoy myself or 'be in the moment' no matter where I was, how cool an event I was attending, who I was with, or what I was doing. All I could think about was what I was go-ing to eat for breakfast the next day, how bad what I had eaten that day was, how much exercise I could get that week, and what new sport or activity I could try, that might magically make me be able to continue my crazy eating behaviors, but still lose weight. Although I could clearly see that my eating and compulsive exercising behaviors sucked, the thought of changing them was very scary for me, because I couldn't imagine how that would possibly work without me ballooning into the 'Goodyear Blimp'.

My journal at the time is filled with re-written, scratched out and edited diet plans that would change each week, and each week I would cryingly, desperately talk to myself in the mirror and solemnly promise myself I would do better this time.

My weight was now fluctuating enormously every single month, depending on what diet or fast I was on. It was incredibly emotionally unbalancing to be fluctuating so much continually. People wouldn't recognize me depending on what month they had met me, and I had to give up modeling and acting for good in early 2003, after I got fired from a job in L.A, partly because of my demanding food requirements and my unbalanced attitude. After getting fired from that last contract, I went on a 3 month long 'mother-of-all-binges' and started feeling increasingly apathetic about whether I lived or died.

Not only was I no longer a glamorous, jet-setting party girl, I was completely unrecognizable from how I used to look. All of a sudden, it felt like the doors to all the VIP rooms had been surreptitiously closed and the 'velvet rope' had been pulled across, with me on the outside of it. My self-esteem, which had become almost completely based on my looks, took a nose-dive. I more or less went into hiding, skittish and paranoid that I would bump into someone who knew "the old me".

Frustrated with the fact that I was becoming so ego-driven and irritable, I decided to take my first 10-day long silent meditation retreat. After that experience, I could never again go back to being quite as superficial and appearance-obsessed as I had once delighted in being, but my path ahead to recovery was still long and winding.

2003 was my last-ditch effort to try anything it took to get thin again. I was getting desperate, and this was reflected in the types of diets and fasts I was trying. For 9 months, I became a raw food vegan (nearly destroying my teeth in the process). As the year went on, the length of time I spent fasting was getting longer and longer. Now really all I could think about was food, weight, eating, exercising and dieting. I was constantly planning where I could get these unusual foods I was eating and how I could get the food as quickly as possible to a private place so I could binge on it. I needed to binge in private, so I found myself digging into baked goods and chocolate in stairwells, toilet stalls, hidden benches inside malls and anywhere else I could get away from the prying eyes of people who dared to judge my huge, sugar-laden feasts.

On my last fast, I had almost lustful cravings for foods that I didn't even like- I daydreamed about all kinds of random foods I hadn't eaten since I was a child. I had thoughts of stabbing and choking myself with food. I was also having nightmares about bingeing on forbidden food and many different nightmares involving food and weight. It was becoming increasingly apparent that I had a serious problem and I started spending time in the eating disorders section at my local bookstore, looking for some answers.

I wasn't anorexic, I wasn't bulimic, so maybe I didn't really have an eating disorder, right? I was still in serious denial. I confided in another 'raw food vegan' friend, who was also a self-professed food addict. But the whole raw foods community seemed a bit like a cult to me, and I was feeling like it might be time to break free.

After the last, really long fast, I had gotten back down to my modeling weight, but as soon as I started eating again, the weight came on incredibly quickly. Within no time I was even heavier than I'd ever dreamed possible and I was freaking out! I started spending time at the local Eating Disorder Center. I remember the first time I spoke to the counsellor there, after I had just finished reading one of Geneen Roth's books. I asked her "Is it possible to do the 'breaking free from emotional eating' plan yet still only eat raw fruits, vegetables and nuts?" It makes me laugh now to think about it- I had such a long way to go.

In January 2004, I embarked on the scariest journey of my life: I let go of all my food restrictions for once and for all. I went from being a vegan, chronic faster, to a junk food junkie overnight. I have never eaten so many chocolates, pastries and baked goods in my life. Although I was taking steps in the right direction, I have to admit that those first few months were the scariest and most miserable in my life. They say that "The only way to it is through it." Well those first few months after taking that desperate, blind leap of faith into 'intuitive eating', I felt like I was groping through a treacherous swamp, desperately hoping that what lay on the other side was worth my daunting journey into the unknown.

Shortly thereafter, I went to a Geneen Roth, 'Emotional Eating' workshop and it was helpful, but I still had so much personal growth and self reflection to do. My face and body were so bloated from all the sugar and salt that I could barely recognize myself and I panicked and decided to go to work and travel abroad for half a year to try to 'get myself together'. Sadly, at a time when I needed support the most, I chose to ostracize myself in a foreign country where I knew no one, and I still told very few friends and family members what was really going on with me. Overseas, lonely and depressed, my only friend was food. I couldn't even get books in English about eating disorders. I was bingeing like crazy and my compulsive exercising was getting out of control, but my metabolism had finally started giving up on me, and I started having to buy clothes in sizes I had never dreamed possible.

Here's a typical journal entry from that time:

March 30/04

"When I first arrived here, I was on a 'one meal a day, starting when I wake up and ending when I go to sleep' meal plan. My eating for the past couple of days

has been very often and large quantities. I see a bit of a pattern: I get excited about following Geneen Roth's Eating Guidelines, and go for it for a few days then for a few days I rebel and binge. It makes me very, very sad and hopeless on the days that I binge. I feel like I'm going crazy. Today is one of those days unfortunately. I know I will look back on this entry one day and cry with empathy for the reality I am living in at this moment. It will change. I know it with every fibre of my being. I think I am trying to rush the process. I can't help it. I want to be happy and free, not lost and confused. I should probably weigh myself soon so I can at least get a reality check. In February I weighed XXX, so I probably weigh XXX now. Please dear God don't let it get higher than that. I want to call Michelle for some therapy talk or e-mail Lisa. I really could use a therapist. Can I find one in a country where no one speaks English? I don't know about the e-mail therapy thing. **Just know that every month you survive is another month closer to breaking free. It takes time."

I had started the very beneficial habit of regularly writing about my feelings in my journal, and that was a step on the road to recovery. But my exercising was getting really extreme. I would force myself to dance for several hours non-stop at the clubs on the weekends, then walk a huge distance across town in the middle of the night, to my boyfriend's house. The next day I would barely be able to walk, but I would never miss a day of either going to the gym or dancing for hours at a time. I loved dancing, but I was at a point where I was risking ruining my favorite hobby by compulsively over-doing it.

I started doing some phone counselling, which was OK, but it didn't feel as helpful as sitting down in a therapist's office. I returned home later that year without having made much too much progress in my recovery, but at least enough time had passed for me to realize that by letting go of my food restrictions, I wasn't going to spontaneously combust, nor would I turn into the 'Goodyear Blimp'.

When I got home, I got a job that I liked, got lots of love and nurturing from my friends, and in my typical pattern, was suddenly re-inspired to lose some weight. The eating disorder books I had been reading warned me to not bother trying to lose weight until I had changed my underlying beliefs and thought patterns, but I didn't want to hear that. I wanted to fit back into my old clothes before they went out of style, damn it! Within a couple of months of moderately watching what I ate, I was fitting into some of my old clothes again and getting lots of compliments. But then things started getting really stressful at my new job and guess what happened? Food came to the rescue! And along with it, came all the pounds that I had pointlessly lost over the last couple of months.

In 2005, I also got into the habit of being addicted to work, and often slept at my office and worked 15-20 hours a day. A pattern of addictive behaviors had become increasingly clear, but I was still unaware of it. My first addiction was binge drinking, then smoking, then bingeing on drugs (although these behaviors didn't happen with enough frequency for me to notice a serious problem). Then I was addicted to getting attention from boys, often kissing several guys per week (or even in one night). I was also addicted to shopping for new clothes with my credit cards, when there was clearly no money in sight to pay the bills when they came. Another addiction was the way I compulsively read entertainment gossip magazines like People and US Weekly from cover-to-cover, every week. My week started revolving around when the next issue would hit the newsstands, although I realized that these magazines were hurting me by feeding into my cycle of body image and diet obsession and pulling me away from my spiritual path with their superficial and shallow messages.

But my favorite addiction, and also the hardest to break, was overeating food. One positive step I was taking was that I regularly spent several hours each month at the Eating Disorder Center, reading, watching educational videos, talking to the wonderful counsellors and writing in my journal. I also went to some therapy sessions with the same counsellor I had phone counselling sessions with when I was travelling. Once my mom even came and that was very enlightening for me, since our relationship has been extremely challenging and she had contributed to shaping a lot of my beliefs and behaviors about appearance, lifestyle, food and weight.

When the project that I had been working on was finally over, I did what I was in the habit of doing: jumped on the next plane to yet another foreign country to get away from all the stress in my life. But unfortunately, in my planning of a relaxing and fun trip abroad, I forgot that I was bringing myself with me. Within a couple of weeks of my arrival, I got mugged, started binging with fervor and more or less had a nervous breakdown, sitting in the middle of the street and bawling uncontrollably.

Out of complete desperation (because, trust me, this was the last thing I wanted to be doing on my exciting trip) I picked up a book about meditation and loving-kindness that a friend had lent me. Again I had the experience that this book held exactly what I needed to hear at that moment. I did a little research about silent meditation retreats and found out that the place that these courses were held was only an hour and a half drive away, and one was starting in less than a week.

I ended up spending more time at the meditation center than I did on the beach that summer, and it was definitely for the best. I have a great deal of respect for any spiritual path, if a person feels it deeply and walks the path with commitment, so I would never say that one path is better than another. All I know is that meditation has been an incredibly grounding and balancing force in my life. Days of meditation in complete silence allowed me to feel like I was taking a step back from myself, and observing my behavior patterns and my history deeply and objectively.

When I returned home in early 2006 I decided to finally join a private eating disorder support group with seven members. It was the first time I had regularly been able to talk openly about my eating disorder. I thought I had to do it on my own for so long, but this group was really helpful in getting everything all out in the open. I started to see the similarities between eating disorders and other compulsive behaviors, addictions and obsessions.

By this time I was meditating every day and I decided to take another ten day, silent meditation course. I still didn't know what I had been running from all these years. Then one day at the meditation center, a link between my subconscious and conscious mind seemed to just click! I had a clear and intuitive memory of myself at around three years old, inseparable from my security blanket and constantly sucking my thumb. I remembered some of the things my mom and I had talked about in counselling. I had reminded her of my father and she had always been callous, belittling and emotionally unavailable to me as a child. I remembered how my sister had taken her cues from my mom and treated me with loathing, criticism and verbal abuse. I remembered how my dad had seemed to love me, but had such unpredictable mood swings that I never knew if I could turn to him for comfort.

Then I thought about my behavior patterns and my addictions over the last several years. Why did it seem like I always had my big binges after getting fired from a job, feeling like someone might me judging me, or feeling nervous and unsure about a challenging situation? Why did I binge after auditions, job interviews or parties? Why did I always refer to myself as a "nervous person"? Why did I jump from one addictive behavior to the next when I began feeling uncomfortable feelings? What was the pattern here!?

And then a huge realization swept over me and tears started streaming down my face as I stood alone in the forest at the meditation center. I realized that, at a very young age, when little day-to-day things would cause me anxiety or confusion, I had no one to soothe me or help me feel safe and nurtured. Therefore, much of my time in my early childhood years was spent in a constant state of anxiety, desperate for a hug or nurturing from my mom, who was never prepared to teach me healthy ways of soothing myself from anxiety. My mom said that I reminded her most of my dad when I cried, so in the moments where I was most in need of solace and consolation, I was greeted with an impassive, blank, cold stare from my mom, which seemed to say "Who the hell are you? Do you really think I could be bothered trying to help you? I wish you were never born." After I graduated from my security blanket and sucking my thumb, I started finding more and more unnatural ways of soothing my anxiety as time went by, when the one thing I was really craving all these years was love and nurturing from my mom.

Finally the truth was clear to me: I had a serious problem with anxiety! It really wasn't about the food at all. I had a huge aversion to ever letting myself feel as vulnerable or afraid as I had as a small child, with no one to soothe me or tell me that it would be all right. Looking back on these memories, I intuitively sensed that I had subconsciously made myself a promise as a child, that when I was big enough to have control, I would never let myself feel that vulnerable or fearful again. My heart ached as I realized that all these years when I had been throwing myself from one guy's arms into the next, what I was truly craving was a reassuring hug from my mom. And unfortunately the one thing I truly wanted was completely impossible to get through my unfulfilling experiences with guys.

I also remembered that although my mom didn't give me emotional support as a child, she had told my siblings and I lots of stories about her glamorous life-style when she was young, beautiful and living in L.A. She talked of how she had met famous people, dated tons of guys and travelled the world.

I looked back on my life.

All of a sudden I realized that although I thought my relationship with my mom wasn't nearly as meaningful as my sister's relationship with her, I was the one who had been mimicking her in so many of my choices as an adult! I also remembered how my mom had been a bit compulsive and hoarding around choco-late when we were growing up. One of the only signs that I got that she loved me was when she would offer to share some of her chocolates with me. And now I was a self-professed "chocolate addict".

These realizations about how I had spent over 20 years acting out an unful-filled dynamic between a mother and child saddened me deeply. But after I had cried out all my tears about it during the next few days, I felt like a ton of bricks had been lifted off of my shoulders. I had read about a woman whose eating disorder had changed almost instantly when she realized that what she had been stuffing down with food all these years was that she was a lesbian. After she came to this realization and started being open with people about it, her eating disorder started to just naturally subside.

I felt the same way when I discovered that my real problem was coping with anxiety. I started opening up to all my friends about my eating disorder and my problem dealing with anxiety. Suddenly I was comfortable mentioning my eating disorder in front of a room full of people, and I made a point of telling any remaining family members or friends who didn't know about my problem.

Over the next few months, through more meditation and soul-searching, I started seeing my problems like layers of an onion that were slowly being peeled back to reveal themselves. When I first began my recovery, I thought my main problem was that I wanted to find a permanent way to lose weight and be attractive. Pretty quickly that layer was pulled away and I realized that what lay beneath that was a dysfunctional relationship with food and body image. Underneath that was a problem coping with anxiety and expressing my feelings. Underneath that was a damaged and emotionally debilitating relationship with my nuclear family from my childhood. Underneath that was a fundamental feeling of unworthiness. And I now believe that after peeling away all the layers and getting to the very core, what remains inside my heart is a feeling that this eating disorder was given to me as a spiritual wake-up call to remind me that I will have a much happier and more harmonious, useful life, when I start living my life to help the community and the greater good, rather than having a self-centered nature, as I had for so many years. But as I continue on this path, things are becoming clearer and clearer each day.

Everything in my life fundamentally changed when I finally got to truly know myself. And what about my eating patterns? Well they changed a lot too. I started respecting and honoring my body in a different way than I ever had before and I started to really enjoy and seek out healthy foods more often than before. There are still times when I emotionally eat but I try not to be as hard on myself about it these days. I stopped going out dancing every night and chose to stay home and read a book, meditate or spend time with friends and family sometimes.

Sometimes I look at my life now and I bemoan the fact that it's not nearly as glamorous or exciting as it used to be, nor do I have a model body any more. In order for me to become healthy, balanced, grounded and well-adjusted, many aspects of my life had to fundamentally change. But these days I am able to feel happy and content with so much less than I used to think I needed to be happy.

My relationships with all my family members and friends are getting much deeper as I open up more to them. I am happy to report that I had a heart-to-heart with my mom and told her that I genuinely forgive her 100% for what happened in the past. I now feel like we are getting closer and closer each day. I feel like I am finally becoming a mature adult, after all these years. My friend told me that when a person gets an addiction, they cease the maturing process at the time they begin their addiction. I can clearly see that I was more mature in my early twenties than

I was when I was in the thick of my eating disorder. And now that I am through it, I feel like my maturity is playing a quick game of "catch up" and all of a sudden I understand a lot of things that I couldn't see before.

I know that life is filled with ups and downs, and that there will be times in the future when life will throw me a curve ball. In a typical week, I seem to go through a wide range of moods: from happy and excited, to lonely, to bored, to feeling disappointed or grouchy. I recently told a friend I met in the eating disorder group "I can't believe how many feelings I have to feel now that I'm not stuffing them down with food, shopping, reading magazines, or any other compulsive, mind-numbing activity!"

It certainly is a big adjustment. But I now have many different tools to deal with my emotions and my anxiety, and I continue to learn more skilful ways of handling and expressing my feelings. I am reading a book at the moment called 'Peace Pilgrim' and when she is asked why people are given problems in their lives, this is her reply: "Constantly enlightenment is being offered to them, but they refuse to accept it. Therefore, they are being taught by problems that are set before them, since they refuse to make right choices voluntarily." If anyone could learn one thing from my story, I hope it would be that getting in touch with your deepest feelings and your inner wisdom is one of the most necessary steps to ending addictions. May we all make peace with our addictive behaviors, and find peace within ourselves.

By N.C., 30. Canada. Disordered Eating for 6 years. In Recovery. Practicing Mindfulness Mediation Daily.

Taking back my Life

By Rachel Beattie, 25. Taunton, England. Former Anorexic, Bulimic, Self-harmer. Recovered.

I could easily sit here and write about how I fell from health to a skeletal mess. How my life went from a meaningful existence to an empty death wish, a mass of despair and nothing to hope for but a quick departure. That would be pointless. How is describing the slow deterioration of a messed up human being actually going to help anyone? Simple answer: it won't. Instead I will explain how it is that I am now sat here, 25 years old, healthy, successful, loved and confident that I will now cope with anything the world has to throw at me. There will be things I will talk about and things I won't mention because some of it I just don't want on paper. It's not fair to those involved or to me. I probably won't even touch on the magnitude of my recovery or even begin to describe the true hell that I had to face in order to be who I am today but I will try.

On a rainy April day in 1998 I sat, 17 years old, jiggling from side to side in a psychiatrist's office wearing tights, skirt, vest, t-shirt, long sleeved top, roll neck jumper and a thick fleece jacket shivering like I had been stood waiting for a bus in the snow for half an hour. To normal people the office was sweltering but to me my bones were literally frozen and radiating cold waves from inside out. I don't remember a word that was said in that room.

Six hours later I was sat in a hospital bed hugging myself; bony knees to chest whilst nurses gave me evil "what are you doing wasting a perfectly good place on the ward?" glares. The only feeling I remember was relief. Stupidly I thought that having medical professionals actually acknowledge my illness would mean that magically I would be free of it. A switch would be flipped and I would eat and be happy with myself as if it was all a bad dream. The reality was about as far away as you could get from that. Nothing had changed except that I now had a whole load of other people to fight against as well.

A nutritionist came to see me. She made me a meal plan. I looked at it and thought how delicious it sounded … for someone other than me. To me it looked like a prison sentence. A death defying feat. A practical impossibility. I stayed in hospital for three weeks. Every day I was weighed. Every day I had my blood taken. Every day I was spoken to like I was a manipulative, naughty little girl. At the time I felt hard done by. Like an innocent party falsely accused. Now I know it was all completely true. The drinks they gave me to build me up went down the sink in their syrupy entirety. The meals I was given stayed in my stomach for approximately 5 minutes until I could get to the bathroom and the rubbish that came out of my mouth about my desire to recover astounded even me. Then I went home to be seen as an outpatient constantly thinking – How the hell did I get away with that?

I remember my first appointment at my counsellor, *June's office. I stepped on the scale at the weight of a nine year old and was promptly told that if I didn't gain weight I would be placed into a unit. As strange as it sounded, even to me, I was more terrified of being put with other anorexics than I was of eating. I knew that my competitive, obsessional personality would spell the end for me in one of those places. I knew I would come up short against others because I didn't think I was a real anorexic. So I listened. I lied. I tried to think about what it would be like to eat what I was being told to and I started to think that maybe I could manage to put on just a few pounds. Just a few mind you.

I was shown a chart. This is my clearest memory of that time. My current weight was pointed to on the bottom of the y-axis. My target weight was shown at the top. That weight seemed like the most ludicrous thing I had ever seen. All I could think of was how fat I would be at that weight. How disgusting and weak I would become. The bizarre thing to me was that at that time I didn't actually think I was fat. I thought I was acceptably thin. I was confused as to why I was being taken seriously as a real anorexic. After all aren't anorexics supposed to think they are fat all the time? Aren't anorexics supposed to think they are humungous blobs when they are actually tiny skeletons? I was sure that wasn't me because my reflection told me on a daily basis that I was reasonably thin. Not skinny by any means but fine.

I was asked to lie down in my underwear on a piece of paper. June got out a big felt tipped pen and drew around my body like you would do to your hand when you are a child. She said it would help me see what I really looked like. I was thinking, "Yeah, whatever you say" because I knew I was going to look fairly thin when she held up the paper. I knew she wasn't going to get the reaction she wanted.

I was wrong. I was so wrong. She held up an outline of a disgusting non-human angular frame with jutting hips, knees, collarbones and I gasped. I gasped and I cried.

June scared me. She told me that she liked my long hair but that I used it to hide my face. She said that when anorexics recover they often cut their hair. She also kept on about how the relationship I was in might not last forever. I didn't want to hear, I didn't want anything to change. I loved my boyfriend. He was my life, my rock, my everything. He stood by me no matter what. I didn't know that seven years later everything June had said would come true. My almost nine year relationship ended, as hard as it was to let go. I treated him badly for a long time and I regret that but I suppose that's how you behave when you aren't yourself.

Over the next few months I was seen twice a week: once to get weighed and discuss my diet and have my weight plotted on a chart, and once to begin to sort the wild misconceptions and strange goings on in my head. Every week before I was weighed I would write down fictitious diet diaries with food that hadn't even passed my lips. I avoided mentioning the other stuff that went into my stomach and didn't stay there. I was starting to drink my strange syrupy nutritional drinks. I didn't mind them because I could lie to myself and pretend they weren't real food. I started to put on a minute amount of weight each week. I was actually, on average gaining less than half a pound but it was enough to keep people happy and I didn't notice it too much. I started eating breakfast cereal in the morning and continued to put on weight.

About four months in, June left and *Lucy took over. For a few weeks I continued to gain weight but then I sort of plateaued. I reached a state of equilibrium where I could manage to eat cereal for breakfast but everything else I ate came back out. I was drinking my drinks most of the time but I stopped gaining weight.

Worried looks were exchanged, hushed discussions about me were had and I was threatened with the unit again. I started to cheat at weigh in sessions and my weight continued to slowly rise (well it did to those who didn't see my real weight on my bathroom scales at home). I fluctuated at this time. I was doing all right and my issues were being talked about but I was still very anorexic and I had pretty much decided that I was quite happy where I was.

I began to have nightmares. I would be staring in the mirror and my teeth would start to ache. My fingers would carefully wiggle a tooth until it came away between them with a sickening wet crack and fell with a clang in the sink. This would then repeat with another tooth and another. I would be left crying, staring at a toothless reflection, desperation and panic welling up inside me like a pillow held over my head too tightly. I pretended to myself that I didn't know what the dreams meant. Who was I kidding? I knew full well what they meant. I was terrified of the damage to my teeth. I knew that throwing a couple of times a day would eventually rob me of my pearly whites. I also knew that the soft aching in my stomach and the constant burning sore throats were not a good sign. Worst of all was my fuzzy swirling head and hot and cold flushes and the heavy breathing like I was going to faint at any moment. I actually started to feel physically worse than I was when I was at my lightest weight.

It began to dawn on me that I really was not well. The fear started to gain momentum because I knew that one day I would be a very wasted, ugly girl if I continued to literally throw my life down the toilet. The thought was like a forgotten chore. The thing you are supposed to remember to do which lurks at the back of your mind and distracts you like a black cloud. I was constantly telling myself, "I'll start eating properly next week, next month, whenever but not today". I felt guilty. I was guilty of ruining my own life. I just didn't know how to stop it. I didn't know if I had the power to face my food fears in order to get my life back. The truth was that as horrid as my life was, it was very simple. I starved, I ate, I threw up and I worked on being a top class student like always. Perfect girl. Secret girl. Everything on the inside girl. An existence like that is very clear and very, very easy. Alarmingly easy.

During my recovery I constantly had to have my blood taken and tested. I remember one occasion sitting in a chair with a needle in my flesh, child's blood pressure cuff around my wasted arm while I looked away. The nurse turned to me and bitterly said, "I used to be nice and thin like you, it just goes to show how things change". I couldn't believe my ears, there I was severely anorexic having blood sucked from my veins and tested because I was so ill and she sat there basically telling me how pleased I should be with my size. This is the hardest thing about trying to recover from being ill. It is like running against a blowing gale, you take a thousand steps but move forwards two like a solitary force against the whole world. Everything is against you. People envy you and don't mind saying it to your face. Everywhere you look there are sickeningly ill looking celebrities proclaiming about this diet and that diet and how healthy they are. We live in a society where to be normal is to be too much. To eat is actually referred to as a sin, "wickedly" rich cake and "devilish" chocolate. No wonder so many people get ill and stay that way. In actual fact, if you do recover from an eating disorder you are likely to belong to a minority of people. Fewer people eat normally than don't. This is the battle we face. You have to be strong to look past it to the heart of life.

I was due to go to university. I wanted to teach. I had always wanted to teach. It was agreed that I could go. I would be transferred to the system in Exeter and would continue to receive treatment. It sounded good to me, a chance to get away and get some breathing space. It was the same old lie I told myself about how now I would actually change and stop being ill just because I was living somewhere else. I really believed that being in a different place meant being a different me. Truth be told I actually wasn't sure that I would last very long as I didn't think I could cope with anything more than my current life but I thought I'd give it a go.

It took a few weeks but I began to love uni. It was so warm. It was a place where the purpose of life was to work. I loved work because it was so rewarding to succeed, someone else judging you, telling you if you are good enough so that you don't have to do it yourself. You don't have to have your own sense of identity if you let someone else decide it for you. My self-esteem was directly correlated with my grades and success. That was part of my problem because I had no identity other than being a perfect student and a committed anorexic. I was a coward to let my life be dictated like that but I couldn't see it at the time.

A month into uni I had an appointment to go and see the new psychiatrist. I readied myself for a good performance and prepared my mind for agreeing to perhaps eat a little bit more.

I had a bit of a shock.

She sat in a chair and I walked in. She looked into me. She didn't look at me. She looked into me and saw the anorexic me who was putting on a false, brave, recovering smile. She smiled at me in a knowing way and asked me to step on the scale. She asked me to do some exercises to show my muscle deterioration. Then I sat down on an orange bobbled chair opposite her. Hundreds of books that had titles referring to eating disorders opposite me caught my eye. She told me she was confused. She didn't understand how the letter she had received from home about me was so positive when I was obviously still very ill and underweight. She worked out a realistic healthy weight for me on a chart. I nearly threw up when she said the numbers. It was more than I'd ever been told to weigh. She told me that I had a very long way to go and that if I really wanted to recover, really truly wanted to be well, then I had to commit myself fully to achieving that weight. I wasn't to agree to it and then put on a few pounds. I had to set my heart on it, strive for it, actively leave my anorexia behind and want to be that weight. She told me that I was to write to her and tell her what I had decided when I had decided it but that if I did decide I wanted treatment I had to mean it and my letter would be kept as proof of my commitment. I left stunned and silent and very afraid.

A few months passed. One night I woke up in a cold sweat feeling shaky. This happened quite a lot but this time it felt different, more real and immediate and like I could actually not wake up in the morning. I often imagined how people would react when they heard about my death. It scared me but what scared me more was the thought that this was going to be my life. If I didn't do something, this was going to be the rest of my life. I would never eat a nice meal and feel no fear. I would never sit on a wooden stool without my bones bruising my thighs through my skin I would never have a comfortable and sound night sleep and worst of all; I would probably never have children.

The next day I wrote the letter.

I was scared when I started to see my new counsellor, *Kate, in Exeter. I felt small and vulnerable and like I was about to have something taken from me. It was the first time I was facing the reality of recovery. She weighed me and started talking to me. She understood. She knew the anorexic me. We didn't talk about what I should eat because she told me that she knew full well that I knew how to put on weight after all when it came to food I really was a pro. We just talked about realistic goals. Tiny steps. How much I would try to gain by the next week. She asked me how I was going to do it. I thought about it and decided I would eat a bit more.

Gradually, I started putting on weight by eating a little bit more here and there. I lasted for four days eating normally and then I started eating too much and the food wasn't always staying where it was put. I thought at the time that I was failing but I wasn't. I was still eating more and throwing up less. It was hard for me because it was at this time that my periods came back. It terrified me because I felt that I really was becoming "normal" but I kept on going. I was meeting my weight goals each week and I actually felt something very strange – FREEDOM. The irony of it was absurd to me; the biggest crime of all – eating, made me feel strong and free. I felt that I could start to shake off my demons, look my illness in the eye and tell her to get lost and leave me alone. One of the most important things Kate taught me was to think of my illness like a separate being, an evil voice. Anorexia was an evil parasite forcing me to do something I didn't want to do. After all you can't fight something unless it is there in front of you to fight and my anorexia was a really nasty piece of work that needed a good kick in the teeth.

As I began to pull away from my illness I wrote "Anorexia" letters. I wrote her sad letters saying how I was going to miss her friendship and help but then they turned nasty and I started telling her how much I hated her. I found this strength inside me. A powerful voice that said no way.

It was me.

My voice.

I was starting to take my life back. I was truly looking at who I wanted to be and saying I don't want this for the rest of my life and I don't care what I have to do to achieve it.

I started working on my fears and my very strange behaviours, which I had never really thought about before. I had so many silly rituals that kept me safe in my head. There were certain times to eat, certain cutlery and crockery to use, certain foods in certain forms and certain numbers of things. I would count out my pieces of cereal one by one in the morning. They had to be complete flakes of cereal. Perfect little wheaty discs. I would eat out of a particular bowl with blue and white checks around the rim and drink from a matching mug. I would have to eat one flake at a time with milk using a teaspoon. Everything had to be ready in front of me at the same time, like I was performing an operation with no room for mistakes.

If I had a sandwich I had to cut it into four exact pieces and eat one piece at a time with exactly one sip of a cup of tea between each bite. If I didn't start eating at exactly the right time the whole lot would have to go in the bin and I would have nothing.

There was also the cleaning, the perfectly wiped surfaces and the spotless floors. I swear that part of me would search out even the tiniest unclean thing just to give me an excuse not to eat. These things sound insane but they allowed me to eat safely. It was like I was given permission by my illness to feed and I liked feeling that I was allowed.

Slowly these behaviours became shackles around my wrists, things that pre-vented me from making any progress. I worked on getting rid of my behaviours. Kate challenged me. She always asked me things like "what would happen if you just poured the cereal into the bowl?". I couldn't reply to that sort of thing because it scared me, even terrified me to the point where I would change the subject. Slowly though, I started to question myself over it. What would happen? I tried it out. Yes I was anxious probably even terrified when I first did it but I did it. I remember the shaking of my hand when I lifted the spoon to my mouth and the milk spilling and dripping down my arm in a trail. But nothing bad happened. It was like a revelation. I started trying other things and again I found that I didn't need to do them. Nothing bad happens if you eat your lunch two minutes earlier than you did the day before. I know it sounds ridiculous but this was my life. My strange beliefs and behaviours. On the one hand I was adamant that I couldn't leave the rituals behind but on the other there was a responsible side to me that knew I had to start acting my age.

I realised that I was actually very childish in a lot of ways. I would behave like a child with everything black and white. Thin or fat, good or bad, success or failure, eat everything in sight or eat nothing. When you grow up you realise there are many shades of grey and living in these shades makes it much easier to get on with your life and not throw a wobbly every five seconds like the Anorexic me did. The grey place is harder but in the long run you know it's for the best.

I started to ask myself why I was scared of recovery. There were many reasons. Anorexia makes you sort of invincible. I was amazing. I could go without eating, I was thin to the extent that people stopped and stared. I pretended I hated it but secretly it made me special. I was worried over. I was mothered. I was constantly watched which made me feel loved and needed and set apart. I was afraid that if I were normal I would be nothing, a grey, non-special, boring old nothing. Of course I didn't admit this to myself at the time because to do that would be admitting I was selfish and needy and I liked to think I was a strong, unbreakable martyr. I started to think about how my recovery would affect people. I realised that everyone would be proud and happy and that the only negative person would be me. There wasn't a single person who would love me any differently and people were always going to worry. I thought that I might be able to have a life again. I wrote down all the things I couldn't do that I would like to be able to like going out for meals and spending time with my friends without worrying about meals and weight and rules and rituals. It all looked quite tempting but also like a very long way away and frightfully scary too. It was like a picture I was looking at that wasn't reality, a parallel universe where I was who I should have been all along.

I continued pondering for a long time. As I pondered I was gradually getting better without even realising it. Slowly I was beginning to eat more. I was eating breakfast and lunch and snacks and only throwing up once a day in the evening. I did weigh more and it scared me at times. Now and then I would get a building panic rising in my chest but I sort of ignored it like I had done to other things for so long. I did well at uni and always got very high marks in everything I did. I loved being there because it gave me the chance to be different because no one there knew who I was when I was very ill. I started to like the way I was treated as normal. I felt like I could have friends and be well and liked for me. It surprised me but I was funny. I was one of the people in my group of friends who made people laugh and was confident. I loved who I felt I could be.

About a year before the end of uni I suddenly made a decision. My time was running out like a train coming up the tracks behind me. I decided I was going to sort my life out once and for all. I went home and threw away all the foods that made me want to throw up. I went to the supermarket and bought the exact ingredients for seven evening meals, lunches and breakfasts. The key here was this; I didn't buy low fat or diet foods. I bought normal everyday things with fat and sugar and calories in them. That night I ate soup and a roll for my tea. I was absolutely terrified but also excited because I thought that maybe, just maybe I could actually do this. Touch wood. After I'd eaten I couldn't sit still. I was so anxious. I kept pacing and rocking. I wanted to get rid of the food so badly. I distracted myself and watched TV. I went upstairs and had a bath (trying to ignore my "whale" belly that wasn't really there). Slowly the feeling of being full went away and I felt ok again. It was like a wave, it built and built like it was going to explode but then it broke and swept out and lessened and calmed. I went to bed that night and couldn't believe I had done it. The next day came and I had something different for tea. Again I watched TV and had a bath and felt ok. I repeated this every day for nine days and ate a normal diet like a normal person. I felt amazing. I was strong. I was successful and I knew everyone would be so proud of me. I treated myself. I bought myself little presents for doing so well.

On the tenth day I ate too much and I didn't keep the food in my stomach. But this time it felt different. It didn't give me anything. I wished I hadn't eaten too much. I didn't like the way it felt to get rid of my food. The need to eat and throw up had left me. It had been part of my life for years and years but now it was gone and all it did was leave me feeling a failure and a waster. The next day I got back up and started eating properly again and I continued to do this for days after that. Every time I felt bad or upset I wrote. I wrote about how I felt and I challenged every negative thought. I looked in the mirror and told myself, out loud, that I wasn't fat. I was thin. I wasn't going to get fat I was just fuelling myself. I was strong and I wasn't going to let anorexia get her way any more. I was a good person who deserved a life.

The next time I saw Kate she was amazed. I recounted what I had been doing and she sat there astounded. I knew what she was going to say before she said it. It was time. It was time to let me go, to let me go and get on with my life. She told me that she knew I would do well with everything I did and that she was so proud of me. I felt my eyes burning and my heart breaking because this was it. It was finally over. I was strong and I was well and I was going to be ok. I was very sad to leave her and to leave the people that had helped me so much but I knew it was time. I mourned my illness and felt a sense of emptiness when I realised I had to finally turn my back on it but I knew it had to be done.

My life switched. I ate pretty much normally from then on. I tried new things. The things that terrified me like lasagne, biscuits, cake and chocolate. It was all alright. I ate it and I was fine. I didn't put on loads of weight. My weight stabilised. I actually ended up weighing between what June and the psychiatrist had suggested. I ate whatever I liked and my weight was fine. I wasn't fat and I felt good. I was happy and I was free. Through my eyes I saw a thinner person now than I had when I was knocking on death's door.

In the time between then and now I have graduated from university with a first class honours degree with two commendations from the Dean. I have a job teaching, which I love and I now have a new relationship where I can't be anything other than normal because the old me has nothing to do with who I am now. I am happy, healthy and successful and looking forward to a full life with whatever I want to do. There are still thoughts that go through my mind. Sometimes I fall a bit but I get back up. Some days I find myself looking back at the temptingly easy life I had but I know that to go back would mean undoing everything and throwing my life away for nothing.

So, I am the unthinkable. I am the success story. Yes it can be done. Even if your head tells you it's hopeless. Even if you slip and fall on the way, you can clamber back up and keep on going. You don't have to live that way forever no matter how trapped you feel. Start to loosen the chains around your wrists and you will eventually wiggle free. I promise. Just have faith in the real you and your ability to take back your life.

By Rachel Beattie, 25. Taunton, England. Former Anorexic, Bulimic, Self-harmer. Recovered.

* Name has been changed to protect person's privacy.

Step by Step

By Christina, 24. The Netherlands. Struggling with an Eating Disorder for 7 years. In Recovery.

I don't believe anorexia is something you 'catch' overnight. I think it's something that develops over a longer period of time, a process, and that whether you get it or not doesn't just have to do with your present; it also has a lot to do with your past. I think in order to deal with anorexia, to beat it and solve it in such a way that it doesn't come back; you need to know what caused it. I don't believe in a single cause that 'makes' you anorexic, however, and I think that the influencing factors are different for everybody.

I tried to write my own story, my own account of what happened to me, when and how I became anorexic. In doing so, a lot of things fell into place. To me, it was helpful to figure out exactly how food came to be such an important part of my life.

When I was younger, I was picked on a lot. I still don't quite know why, exactly, but I was an outsider from the get-go. I didn't have any friends; I was ignored and beaten up a lot. When I was eight, the situation got out of control, and I had to switch schools. Things were a bit better at my new school, but I was still an outsider. This was due, in part, to the fact that I was good at school. Everybody thought that because of that, I must feel better than anyone else. In fact, the opposite was true. I always felt less than anyone else; after all they were always picking on me and thus made it clear how they thought I was pretty worthless. At home things weren't too great either. My family (mom, dad, younger brother and younger sister) has always been very close, but because of all the trouble at school I wasn't an easy kid to deal with. From the time I went to school until I was about twelve, we were constantly butting heads. I generally felt bad, and that was hard on me and everybody else. Thinking back to this time, I remember it as being pretty much awful, but I know there were a lot of happy moments too. I fondly remember family holidays, family dinners and Saturday nights...

As a toddler, I had been a problematic eater, but I had long gotten past that. I didn't have any problems with eating or with my weight at that time. I have always been small, and for a long time I was able to eat whatever I wanted, without gaining weight. Not that I was paying any attention to that, my appearance didn't matter to me back then.

After moving to another city, things got better both at school and at home when I went to high school. I was picked on less and less, even though the first two years weren't exactly terrific. When I was fourteen, things started to get interesting. I made some friends, and we spent lunch breaks together. I wasn't exactly popular, and I didn't have too much self-confidence, but I wasn't bullied anymore. I felt good, accepted by at least some people. For a long time I hadn't paid any attention to how I looked, it was useless anyway because my peers disapproved no matter what. When I had my first crush, that changed. I started paying more attention to my appearance and felt it was at least somewhat important that I looked good. I was still eating regularly, though, and I didn't worry about my weight, since it pretty much stayed the same anyway.

My eating problems started when I was seventeen. I was really stressed out. It was my final year of high school, and there was a lot going on. There were papers to write, homework to do and exams to study for. A couple of friends and I were planning to have a party to mark the end of our high school career, and there were a lot of activities going on at school. Also, I was feeling quite insecure about going to university. After being at the same school for years, I finally felt pretty safe there, and I didn't have a clue as to what university would be like. I had picked my major, but I wasn't sure about my choice, even though my parents supported me in it. I worried about being in this new city without knowing a soul, studying a subject I wasn't sure I wanted to study. I wondered if people would like me, and if I would be able to do it at all. I was terrified that I might lose touch with my friends, and I knew I wouldn't see the guy I had a crush on at all anymore. At that time, things weren't so great between my mom and me either, typical teen problems I suspect. In addition to this I was nervous about a summer job my dad had gotten me, and about going to see my granddad in Florida, because the relationship with him had been rather strained in the past. All these things made me feel like everything was spinning out of control!

Around the beginning of spring, I started to watch my weight, as a kind of distraction. I was relatively okay with my weight; I just didn't want to gain any. Or so I told myself. At first it wasn't even really like a diet, it just gradually became one. It started with me not having a cookie every single time one was offered. I also stopped using butter on my bread, since I had never really liked it anyway. I was simply trying to watch what I ate, but I gradually started eating less and less. It made me feel good. After a while I started working out in secret. It gave me a huge rush to be able to wear myself out like that. One time, I guess I overdid it, because my feet hurt for weeks, after that I didn't work out much anymore. Even though I knew I was eating less than I should, I wasn't worried. It was no big deal. I even had a minimum that I felt I should eat each day. I had it all under control. Or so I thought.

After I graduated, I went to Florida with my brother, to spend three weeks with my granddad. By itself, it was a great experience, but in light of the not-so-good past relationship it wasn't easy. I remember him telling me I had better watch my weight, or I would get fat. Afterwards, it turned out it had been his idea of a joke; in fact he had probably meant just the opposite. If I hadn't been in trouble already, I would never have cared so much, but it did really hurt me at that time. I already felt really fat, because there were a lot of fat people around and there was all this food available. I didn't want to eat too much of it. My brother noticed at that time, and commented on it. But since I didn't get the chance to weigh myself, I feared I would have gained loads of weight by the time I went back home if I didn't watch myself, so I kept close tabs on what I ate. During that period, too, it was a distraction. Whenever I felt bad or out of control, which was quite often, I concentrated on what I would or wouldn't eat.

I started at university in September. I enjoyed it, although it took some getting used to. It was a small and intimate group of people and I gradually felt better about it. However, my mom was starting to let me know she was worried about how little I was eating. I didn't agree with her assessment, I just didn't eat as much as she did, what was wrong with that? A part of me knew what the dangers were, but I promised myself I would be careful, and I was convinced I didn't have a problem.

Just when I was starting to feel like I belonged at university, my dad became ill. Pretty much overnight we found out he had cancer. Then of course, nothing was the same anymore. My mom didn't know how to deal with the situation. She leaned on me a lot, told me everything, how bad it was for her, how scared she was... I was the one having to take responsibility, be strong, encourage her and comfort her when she cried. She felt she had to tell everybody who was willing to listen what was going on. By telling her story, she got to vent and she got attention, which she needed desperately. I needed attention myself, of course, it was hard for me too, but I wasn't somebody who easily opens up and talks about her feelings. Also, I found it was very difficult for somebody who hasn't been in a situation like it to understand what it feels like, so I didn't really try to talk to anybody. I couldn't talk to my mom either, though. Whenever I tried to tell her how I felt, she would start crying, and then it was up to me to comfort her. This made me feel very lonely and neglected. I hated how everyone kept asking me how my mom was holding up, and forgot to ask how I was doing. Also, even though it was in part my fault because I tended to keep my emotions to myself, I was angry with my mom for getting so much attention and not giving me any, for leaning on me so much that I didn't get the chance to feel my own pain.

My mom started eating less during that time. This happened without her even trying very hard. She has been slightly overweight for a long time, and has been dieting on and off for as long as I can remember. This time, however, she actually lost some weight, in part due to stress. Her friends noticed this and paid attention to it. I guess this might have made it more important to her. She started to talk about it a lot, kept repeating how her clothes had gotten too big for her, and she could fit mine, and how much weight she lost. She would say this several times a day, and because I was already having trouble eating, I hated how she emphasized her weight loss. It felt like a personal assault, that what she meant was that I was as 'fat' as she was. I felt like what she wanted more than anything was to be thinner than me, that it was some kind of contest. I became convinced that the worst thing that could happen was her becoming thinner than me. The whole thing became a distraction, whenever my dad was doing worse and my mom started dumping all of her problems, worries and feelings on me, I thought about not eating and losing weight and felt in control. It was also a way to voice my anger. I was angry with my mom for letting me down, for getting attention when I didn't, for not being there for me... but at the same time I felt it was unreasonable of me to feel this way. By eating less I could punish her without risking a direct confrontation. It was like a scream for attention. Not eating was trying to regain some control when everything around me was spinning out of control. I didn't feel in control of my world and all that was happening in it, but by not eating I could at least control my weight, and myself, or so I thought. In reality, the anorexia was controlling me.

By January of 2000 my brother and my mom started making these jokes about me eating so little and becoming so thin. In jest, they even called it anorexia. I didn't like that and felt it was totally unjustified, but in a way it was also a rush, some form of attention of course, which I needed so desperately. I had figured out calorie counting by then and kept a precise record of what I ate, trying to limit my intake as much as I possibly could.

By March I realized it was increasingly controlling my life and I didn't want to be so obsessive anymore. I understood I wasn't doing well and wanted to quit, meaning that I still wanted to eat little and lose weight, but without being obsessive. I didn't even realize that eating that little was a big part of the problem. And I couldn't pull it off. By May I had started reading books on anorexia. Until that time I didn't have a clue that I had a real problem, but I recognized a lot and started to see that I was at risk. Still, I was convinced I had it all under control. I didn't realize I was already anorexic.

Meanwhile, my dad was doing worse every day. We still had hope in the beginning, but after the operation in January had failed, things went downhill from there. My dad died in June of 2000. My mom fell apart. It was like she wasn't even there anymore, she did the craziest things, and I was the one who had to keep things together. During all this, anorexia was my escape from reality.

It was always there, it controlled my life completely. I tried to eat as little as I possibly could without anybody noticing there was a problem. I was convinced that all my mom wanted was for me to get fat and I didn't want to let her win. My weight totally determined my mood, gaining an ounce got me depressed, losing an ounce made me feel exhilarated -for a short while, because I kept wanting to lose more. The 'goal' kept shifting downward. I didn't have time to think about anything else, for example how much I missed my dad. As soon as I felt I was getting upset, I started summing up what I ate, calculating how many calories I still had 'left' and what I would have to eat. What saved me, in retrospect, was that I was more or less forced to keep eating dinner. I was terrified that my family would find out about the anorexia, so I never dared skipping dinner for fear they might realize what was going on and try to stop me. This kept me from losing too much weight, even though I was underweight.

The fact that I was eating so little had a lot of effect on my body. I was cold all the time. I felt hungry and empty almost constantly and was lightheaded. I was always tired, but in a way I felt energetic as well. My nails kept breaking and my hair looked awful. My weight totally determined my mood, I was terrified that if I ate one bit too much, I would start gaining weight and this wouldn't stop until I was really really fat. It was always on my mind. The first thing I thought when I woke up in the morning was what my weight would be and how much I would or wouldn't eat that day. I lived from 'meal' to 'meal' and calculated the amount of calories in everything I ate at least a dozen times. Having to eat something unexpectedly, when I couldn't get out of it, I panicked. Knowing I would have to eat something extra, I compensated twice the amount of calories, just in case. I drank as much water and tea as I could, but that didn't make me feel less hungry. In a way it even felt good to be hungry, it was a confirmation of the fact that I was indeed eating too little and therefore would lose weight. Feeling hungry became an addiction. As long as I got to stick to my schedule, I was all right, but the slightest deviation caused terror, and getting fat seemed like the worst thing that could ever happen.

I tried to stop the obsession in July, September and October. A part of me knew that what I was doing was really dangerous and that my thoughts were off, but I still couldn't do it. For a long time I didn't even really want to quit, I just didn't want to feel desperate anymore. I did want to feel better, but I didn't want to eat more and I certainly didn't want to gain weight. That's impossible; you can't recover from anorexia without reaching a normal, healthy weight, but I didn't know that at the time. After a while, I wanted to quit for real, but I was certain I never could. I couldn't imagine a life without anorexia, what it would be like to just eat something without feeling guilty. I didn't have a clue how to fight it. I didn't want to lose it either, in a way, it had become my way of controlling the world, my safe base, my distraction to prevent me from thinking about my dad or anything else that might upset me. What was I to do if I lost that? For a long time I even thought I was just making something out of nothing, calling it anorexia when there was really no problem. But more and more I recognized myself in the stories on the Internet and I started to realize I did in fact have an eating disorder.

Study-wise, I had switched majors by then, my first choice turned out to be not quite right for me. This new subject was fun, only I was bored. I had too much time to spare, so I used this time to think about not eating.

By November my mom said she wanted to talk to me. She asked me if I was afraid to gain weight. Even though I had promised myself I wouldn't tell her any-thing, I did admit to that. I didn't let her in on how bad I really was doing, but I did acknowledge I didn't want to gain any weight. She said she felt I wasn't eating enough, but I told her she didn't eat much more herself, which she did admit to. She also said she felt there was some sort of competition going on, which I denied. She had me promise to eat more, and she promised to eat more herself. I did prom-ise, but I didn't mean it. On the contrary, I did worse than ever. Still, my mom complimented me on my eating not much later. I was really proud of myself.

My relationship with my mom was really bad by then. We were always butt-ing heads. We weren't fighting, exactly, but we were assuming things about one another, and acting on them without checking if they were true. I constantly felt like she was mad at me, disappointed in me. My younger sister was 'on my side', telling me what my mom was saying about me, and I believed what she told me. In retrospect, I don't think she meant to lie, but hearing things second-hand is always different, and I didn't know the context in which those things were said. In January of 2001 I had an ear operation. From then on, things were a little better between my mom and me. I was disappointed in her, though, for not being there for me and leaning on me like she was, and for not seeing how much trouble I was in, even though I was the one trying to hide it from her at all costs. Around that time I stopped getting my period, my body didn't have enough reserves for it. It didn't bother me at first, I had never liked it anyway, and besides, I was too preoccupied with not eating. My body was letting me down, I didn't feel well, but I still didn't think it was serious. I had read these horrible stories of anorexics weighing close to nothing, I wasn't like that. I was still eating after all: it could be so much worse. In reality I was doing pretty badly. A lot of people make that same mistake; they think that as long as you're not completely emaciated and in the hospital, you don't have anorexia. But it's not about being fat or skinny; it's about what's going on inside of you. There are plenty of people who are very thin, but don't have anorexia. There are also many anorexics that aren't all that thin. You can't always tell from the outside.

By April, I finally realized what I was doing. I knew that I could really damage my body. I understood that the fact that I didn't get my periods anymore was a bad sign; it could have serious consequences. I might become infertile. I really want to have children, some day. I saw that I wasn't just destroying my present; I was also ruining my future and that of my potential children. It was only getting worse. And even though it got worse slowly, both my body and my mind were falling apart. I realized I had two choices: keeping this up and dying, or fighting it and living. I didn't want to die. I was afraid. That's when I decided it had to end here.

This didn't mean I was 'normal' from one day to the next. Things all got better gradually, and it was anything but easy.

I slowly quit counting calories, which had become an addiction. I started to realize that my mom is not me, and that her being fat or skinny doesn't change me at all. My body was doing better as well. I wasn't cold all the time anymore, I wasn't dizzy anymore, I felt stronger, and my thinking was kind of back to normal. I got my period back fairly quickly, by the end of May, and even though I hated it and it made me feel like I had gained way too much weight back, I was also proud of it. I went back from weighing more than twice a day to only once a week. Also, I started eating more, a little bit at a time. At first I didn't have a clue as to what was normal. Then I got hold of an eating list, like a guideline as to how much 2000 calories a day really is. I tried to follow this schedule for a while, and felt much better, only I felt it was a bit much. So I went back to eating less than what was on the list, because I didn't feel I needed quite so much. Without really noticing at first, however, that was my first step backwards.

There were several causes for my relapse, for example the fact that I had nothing to do and the fact that I got a tooth-infection, which gave me a perfect excuse to skip meals. Then there was my mom, who went on a diet again, including pills and skipping meals, which was and still is a huge trigger for me. I found myself again paying a lot of attention to how much she ate, trying to stay just under that, or at least making sure she didn't know I was eating more than her. It made me feel really weak whenever I ate more than she did, so I ate less. The fact that the self-help group I had applied to by then wouldn't start for another three months didn't exactly help either. At the time I applied, I didn't do so because I felt I was doing badly, I simply wanted help to overcome those final roadblocks, take the final steps. After all, the practical things like weighing and counting aren't the real problem, I had dealt with those, it's the thoughts and feelings that are the hardest to control. However, once I went to a few introductory meetings, I realized I wasn't doing as great as I thought… but also that most of the other girls were doing worse. I think that if the actual group had started right that moment, I would have been okay, but since I had to wait a few months, it was a trigger for me. I felt that if only I lost some weight before we got started, it wouldn't matter so much if they told me to gain weight. It was stupid. I wasn't aware of it at the time. It just happened, but I also let it happen.

During that summer, I got a lot worse. I lost more weight then I ever did, I was more preoccupied with counting calories than ever, I spent every free moment planning my food, I panicked at every meal. I did realize I was doing worse, but I just thought: I have to hold out a few more weeks. Perhaps I felt that at least now I still could count calories, weigh, obsess, use it as a distraction, whereas once the group started, I would have to let go of all of it. All of the progress I made since April year was lost. And that was a real shame!

When the group finally started in September of 2002, however, I started doing better again. I have to say that it helped me a lot to talk to people who knew what I meant, not having to explain why I did something. It also helped to have somebody 'checking up on me', somewhere to go every week to vent.

I started a website when I started recovery, and it has also been a real support through all of this. It got me into contact with others, some doing better than me, some doing worse. It helped me, being to tell my story, and listening to other people's stories. Since nobody knew about my anorexia for three years, I didn't talk to anybody about it for a long time. That was my own choice; I was and am afraid that whenever I tell somebody, the relationship will really change. I am afraid I will always be watched and judged by the people that know about it. That's why it was nice to be able to talk anonymously over the Internet. By now, some of my friends know which is a relief – most of the time. Nothing really changed, they are all great about it, believe and accept it because they care about me. The fact that nobody knew had become like a safety net to me, if I didn't make it, I could always get back to not eating and nobody would be the wiser. I had to get rid of that idea, for my own safety. And of course I really wanted to talk about it; too, I wanted to share. When you have a secret like this for three years it becomes huge, and seems almost surreal. It was such a relief to get it off my chest.

Shortly after I started the self-help group, my family found out about my eating disorder as well. I had been a little less secretive for a while, sort of hoping they would figure it out, and my recent weight loss hadn't gone unnoticed either. I was thinking about telling my mom, but before I found the courage to do so she figured it out on her own. In a way, it was a huge relief, not having to hide it anymore, not having to scheme and pretend and lie. It felt right to be able to share this part of me with my family as well. However, we all needed to readjust to the situation, and we went through some awfully stressful weeks. My mom didn't and still doesn't understand and made that abundantly clear. I also felt a lot of pressure, I felt watched and judged. Also, I felt guilty. Time and again my mom emphasized that the situation was very hard on them. Of course I know that's true, and if I could have prevented that I would have. But I didn't just decide one day that I would be anorexic, it developed gradually. It's hard for all of us, but even though my mom might not agree, it's hardest for me. Things got better slowly, and right now we're at the point where we can discuss it if necessary, although we don't often do so.

After finishing the self-help group, I joined a relapse-prevention self-help group in September of 2003 until the summer of 2004. I found it really helped me to be able to talk about what was on my mind without having to explain every little detail. There was a lot of acceptance and respect in this group, and I found that it made things a lot easier for me.

Since then, things have been up and down. Sometimes I do really well; sometimes I don't do so well. But one thing remains: my determination to never let things go too far anymore. Before, I always wanted to lose one more pound. Now, if I find myself losing too much weight I make sure I gain it back. Weight gain still scares me, though, and I have no intention of gaining more. I am at a healthy weight right now and that is where I want to stay. My eating is much better. At times I don't care at all, and then there are times -usually stressful times- where I find I do care and I watch what I eat a little more. Generally I make sure I eat enough to keep my weight and energy levels constant. I eat three meals a day and three snacks. I go out to dinner occasionally.

However, I don't want to call myself recovered at this point. I'm still recovering. I'm not saying I will never reach 'recovery', but I do know I'm not there yet. There are still things that would need to change, but at this moment I am happy with the way things are. I'm healthy; eating well, feeling good… those last few things are for a later time to deal with. However, I made my choice and I'm not going back. My life is so much better now than it was before.

By Christina, 24. The Netherlands. Struggling with an Eating Disorder for 7 years. In Recovery. For more information, visit Christina's website at **http://www. geocities.com/spacey_christina/**

perfectly imperfect...
that's me.
years and years of pleasing leave you nowhere
and waiting...for the day you can wake up
and see that your life is worth more...

> *i am more than a number on a scale*
> *or the size of my clothes.*
> and **i** am more than a statistic

i am a survivor.

and **i** am more than one of the lucky ones...

today, i have the tools to fight that bondage.
the difference is not that it is easier
but that i have seen and felt the beauty
that each moment of recovery has to offer me.

> she is still as cunning as ever
> she still knows all my weaknesses
> and she still waits, patiently, in the shadows
> hoping for an opportunity
> to once again capture.

but...

the one who fights for me is far stronger...

> **He** uses my weakness for His glory.
> **He** molds my mistakes into true beauty.
> And **He** heals my brokenheartedness.

and He gives me Redemption and Humility.
the chains of rape, abuse, and self-destruction are broken...
and i am freed.

> free to be me. *perfectly* imperfect.

By Amanda Travers Bell, 21, married. Nashville, Tennessee, United States. Anorexia, Bulimia, and Binge Eating for 8 years. Depression, Self-Mutilation, Codependency, Cocaine Addiction, Survivor of Rape and Abuse. In recovery for over 2 years, and getting stronger everyday! Praise the Lord!

I am Beautiful for ME!

By Michelle, 31. Vancouver, British Columbia, Canada. Restricting and Bingeing for 12 years. Recovered.

I cannot remember when I really started to dislike my body…but I believe the process began when I started developing breasts. I wanted to hide them, like many young girls possibly, and did not like the attention they brought even after hiding them as best I could. I would wear super long t-shirts that were so baggy you could fit two of me in there. It didn't matter; I still got honked at by passing vehicles, which I just hated. Why won't they leave me alone?!

Once I entered into high school it became all about comparisons. I felt terribly insecure by the beautiful women I saw and how slight they all seemed to be, and how popular they were as well. I didn't have a delicate frame like they had and was extremely unhappy with myself. Nothing looked chic, or cool, or the way it was supposed to look… basically the way it looked on them, when I tried it on in the store. I stayed away from buying any form fitting clothes, because that would just bring me negative attention! I wanted to look "pretty" and sexy but didn't want to be ogled at by men! They never seemed to look at my face as it was, so the last thing I wanted to do was draw their eyes elsewhere even more. I felt torn inside, hate for my body the way it was but at the same time if I had a wonderful body, men would be even more interested. What I really wanted was to stop feeling so lousy about myself every time I looked at a magazine in the store and so many of the girls at school. I figured that meant looking like them.

My mum would try to console me, telling me I am big boned but yet my wrists are tiny!! She would also tell me I was born with more padding around my hips, and that's just the way I will always be. I hated hearing that, to me she was saying you will always be a big girl. My dad would talk about how great it is for women to have big strong legs, and pat my leg like I had just that. I felt worse.

It wasn't until I experienced mono one summer when I was 14 that I realized the joys of losing weight. Mono hit me hard, I couldn't eat anything but liquids and I ended up losing a good amount of weight. I was thrilled!! I remember getting out of the hospital bed, walking around and feeling so light! It wasn't about feeling unwell or getting better, it was pure excitement to try on clothes I had out grown and I did just that.

From then on it became more of a pre-occupation in my mind. I joined a woman's only gym to keep the weight off and went regularly. I was enjoying feeling fit and strong but what I was really hoping for was more weight loss and a big drop in my body fat percentage. I went to the gym on a regular basis for about a year or so before it closed down. I joined a co-ed one shortly after but I barely went at all. The atmosphere was uncomfortable to me, it seemed again to attract men's attention and I found myself hating the women who had sculpted bodies. I gave up and would eat in my hatred for myself, for what I will never have. I binged when I ate, eating tons of starch and sweets, the most comforting foods and then I would feel even worse about myself and the cycle kept repeating over and over.

Before I left high school I started walking an hour every evening, I just needed to get out of the place I was staying and to my surprise I lost a lot of weight yet again. I was thrilled! This benefited me when I started working at a ski hill, in the gift shop, after graduating from high school. I found I was quite popular with men. I still couldn't stand being ogled but I enjoyed men's interest in talking with me and I seemed to get asked out quite a bit.

Shortly after, I went overseas to work but the situation was terrible. I was isolated out in the middle of no where and fell into a depression. The food binge-ing started and when I came back home I was the heaviest I had ever been yet. I wouldn't go out, I wouldn't look for work, I was very depressed. All I could do was eat and sleep it seemed. In desperation I joined a weight loss centre and bought a stair master so I didn't have to go out to exercise. The food I had to buy from the centre was disgusting and expensive and I felt faint from the few amount of calories I was allowed in the rationed out, pre-made boxed portions. Yes, I lost weight, but I didn't feel good. I remember my dad seeing me on the street after I had lost a fairly significant amount of weight and commenting how good I looked, reinforcing to me I look better when I weigh less. I also got similar remarks from others I knew. It made me feel worse to hear their praise in connection with weighing less. That was the last thing I wanted.

Shortly after returning from overseas, I moved out to share with my best girl friend. Together we became obsessed with losing weight. She, already being skinny, thought she was fat which made me feel even worse as I weighed at least twenty pounds more than her. We weighed ourselves at least once daily, sometimes a few times a day. It seemed like a competition, when she lost weight

I vowed I would eat even less. I continued to binge on food when I broke down in between, always hiding it from others and feeling worse about myself after, experiencing pure shame and disgust.

My life was all about trying to lose weight and dieting and then a few years later it became dependent on it. The first guy I fell in love with dumped me in an ugly manner. I found out he made a bet he could get this other woman into bed with him. I was absolutely devastated. I was 21 at the time and we had seriously dated for about a year and a half. I became severely depressed, failed all my university courses which was horrific but I couldn't study let alone go to the same university as him, and lost a great amount of weight. I had NO appetite. Immediately others gave me positive feedback when they saw the weight loss. In fact I ran into a woman I had gone to high school with who reacted by saying, "You look so good being thin! So much better!" It just fed into me not being good enough as I usually am… how I have always been.

I scrutinized my body numerous times in the mirror throughout the day, measuring, weighing, pinching, and trying on smaller clothes to see if I now fit into them. I was obsessed and gaunt looking. I didn't like the look of my bones protruding but I still saw so much extra weight to lose. My mum was very worried about me and said I had a problem, and the more concerned she was, the more I took from it. I thought it must be working! I must be losing more weight than I had before! I knew I had, but her voiced concern made me feel proud of what I had accomplished with my weight loss; after all it was really showing now! By the time my appetite started to return I was fret with worry that I would gain it all back and starved myself purposefully now, writing down everything I had ingested to look at just how much I was eating! It seemed to be an awful lot. At this point, I also attempted purging, thinking that's the way to go, that's the answer! I was unsuccessful when I tried, and wondered how women do it so it works.

My family also gave me mixed messages. My mum started pulling out old clothes that used to fit her when she was tiny and young and wanted to see if they fitted me now, and told me how nice I looked in them. My Grandma told me I needed to gain weight but then also thought I looked lovely in my mum's old clothes. It was typical. All my life I had received mixed messages from my family around food and weight. Either told I have gained weight and need to watch it, but please take this second, better yet third helping of food even when I've been completely full, or told I need to gain weight, I look sickly but then complimented for how nice I look being thinner. Crazy making.

I couldn't continue to starve myself successfully with my full appetite back and my biggest fear came true. I binged and binged and binged! I couldn't stop.

I felt like crap, I looked like crap. I gained a large amount of weight, topping the highest I had ever been by 30 pounds! The depression carried on. I attended two support groups for a session each but I didn't feel like I fit in. It seemed I wasn't fat enough for one of them or thin enough for the other to truly belong. I couldn't even classify myself. I wasn't anorexic as I binged, and I wasn't a true compulsive overeater as I starved myself in between. I felt like a failure, I wasn't even capable of getting an eating disorder right! My inability to purge being another failure.

I attended meetings at another type of weight loss centre twice in the years following. The first time I stopped going after I learned how their program worked and did it on my own at home. I hated being weighed in at their centre; it was a humiliating process to me. Women in their spandex, taking off all their jewelry, shoes, even their hair bands so they could weigh less on the scale!! And it didn't matter if I had lost weight when I weighed in, it was never enough. Worse though was if I had gained weight, I felt like a complete failure. What's the point of try-ing!? I didn't want to be like these women, so desperate! I felt like a cow waiting in line to be branded.

I was successful with weight loss both times with the centre, but gave up their eating plan after a number of months. I didn't want to carry on being obsessed about every item I put in my mouth, as you can't help but be when writing down your food intake. In between the two sets of times I joined, I carried on bingeing in secret when upset, which seemed to be daily. Everyone thought I ate so healthy and such small portions; they had NO idea what I really did when no one was around. Whether it meant splurging in the car, waiting before going home to stuff myself with sweets and fatty foods, or in the bathroom. I would hide chocolate and other foods where it wouldn't be found and then eat it as soon as I possibly could. The feeling inside was pure disgust for myself all the time. I felt like a gross person, feeling terrible about my secret that would horrify others if they ever knew just how much I had binged on, or worse caught me!

It wasn't until shortly after when I got a dog that I became a happier person. I was attending college taking a full time course load and walked him usually once a day (my boyfriend walked him the rest of the time). I had always wanted a dog and having him to pet and love at home was therapeutic for me. I was still strug-gling with my weight but I plateaud for a number of years during this time. I con-tinued to eat when not hungry but it was in smaller quantities and less frantic.

When I graduated from my college program, I began to lose weight rapidly. It scared me. It was so rapid and not a result of anything I was doing to try and lose weight. I was losing a dress size a week it seemed and couldn't keep up with my clothes. I went through all the sizes I had worn to a point at which I had to buy new clothes, smaller in size then when I had no appetite after the break up. I went to the doctor to have blood tests done. It made no sense, I had always had to work with ALL my effort to lose weight in the past and now I was doing nothing and it was pouring off me. The doctor didn't find anything wrong and thankfully my weight plateaud. I actually gained back about 15 pounds after a few months, very gradually, and have been the same weight ever since. It has been almost 3.5 years ⊠.

I attribute my success with my healthy weight to a few things. I am more in touch with my emotions. I recognize that I do at times feel down, but eating more does nothing for me. I instead talk with friends or write my thoughts out. I also take action if I'm unhappy with something in my life and wanting change, after all no one else will take care of me but me!

The other enormous contribution in my life has been my dog; he is the greatest love of my life! He keeps me healthy and I have to go out and walk him, rain, sun, or snow! Prior to him, exercise was something to do to lose weight, not to be healthy, social, or responsible for something else other than me. I feel blessed to have him in my life. Recently, after separating from my boyfriend, I became worried that the change in my schedule with the dog would cause weight gain. You see I now share him with my ex boyfriend, so I have him every other week. I am proud to say that I continue to go for a walk daily, even when I don't have my dog and want to continue regardless of the weather or how busy my day is.

The other factor that has kept me at a healthy stable weight has been my relationship with food. I never say I can't eat that! It is no longer about keeping something off limits, or labeling foods bad, but instead balancing out my intake of sweet / high fat foods. It has come naturally. I never feel deprived, never feel like I am punishing myself nor do I have to say no to what I want to eat. The struggle has completely ceased with that.

The remaining area that I am continuously working on is my body image. I am taking an active role in building some muscle in my body. Yes I have stretch marks all over my hips, my thighs still have inches of fat to grab onto, as well as my abdomen and butt. And yes, I have cellulite on my legs and butt, BUT I am at a good weight for myself and I am building muscle to feel better about my body. I have found that individual exercise works well for me as I can't compare my body to other women's. Intellectually I realize women in gyms may have been working on building muscle for years but psychologically it doesn't matter when I see them, I still tend to judge myself more harshly if I am around them and get down on myself. So, I have learned when I don't compare myself I am the happiest. As I am aware of this, I don't look at women's magazines; a recipe for self-judgment with the air brushed under weight models! And talking about weight, my scale is now kept at the bottom of a box of toiletries, and I pull it out maybe once a year just out of sheer curiosity.

I had not worn a bathing suit or a tank top since I was in elementary school, but last summer I took the plunge and started wearing tank tops and bought myself two pairs of board shorts and bikini tops to wear in the water. The main thing is doing what I want to do and feeling comfortable doing it. I don't want my body image to hold me back from experiencing life anymore and have met more women like myself since I have become more aware. When I am ready, one day I will visit the local nude beach and experience life without clothing. Until then, I continue to celebrate what I have achieved and what I do have. I have found it fulfilling to take tasteful photos of myself, enjoying the curves and skin I own ▨. I am more then my thighs, butt and abdomen. I love my full lips, my telling eyes, my elegant neck, my strong shoulders, my chest, my long arms and yes, even my round hips. But more then anything I love who I am, I shine from the inside out! My soul cannot be captured by my appearance!

Appreciate yourself for what you do have, the rest will come. And remember, you are loved by us all!

hugs

Michelle

By Michelle, 31. Vancouver, British Columbia, Canada. Restricting and Bingeing for 12 years. Recovered.

BIG AND BEAUTIFUL

I am beautiful,
and I don't care what you think about me.
My body may not be perfect,
but I have strength in personality.
Too many people like me,
let people like you bring them down.
Well I won't stand for it,
not ever and not now.

We are all different.
We come in all shapes, sizes, and colors.
No one is inferior or better than another.
So what makes you think,
you have the right to criticize me?
If you don't like me,
you are welcome to leave.

I may not look like barbie.
I may not look good in a bikini.
I may not be able to wear a size five.
I may be a little round in the middle,
and have thunder thighs.
But when I look in the mirror,
I know I like what I see,
Because I can appreciate the uniqueness,
that makes me
me.

By Tiffannie Brinkhaus, 25. Minnesota USA. Overeating Disorder brought on by
Depression. In Recovery.

Fallen Angel:
Claiming My Freedom from a Chronic Battle with an Eating Disorder

By Jessica, 26. Houston, Texas USA. Suffered from COE (Compulsive Overeating) turned Anorexia turned Bulimia turned EDNOS (Eating Disorder Not Otherwise Specified) - total of 12 and a half years. 7 time Relapse-Survivor (from the year 2000 to 2005). Finally Fully Recovered! Childhood Sexual Abuse and Rape Survivor. Recovered Cutter. Diagnosed with Mental Illness. Symptom Free from Mental Illness for 1 year!

My name is Jessica, and My 26th birthday is in two weeks (April 26th). They say that's your "Golden Birthday" - when your age and the date of your birthday is the same. It's supposed to be extra special. And this year it will be! The best birthday gift I have ever given to myself is that I can finally say I am recovered from an eating disorder. I truly never, ever thought I'd live to see my 26th birthday (and at times I wasn't sure I wanted to).

My "story" begins early in my childhood, at 7 years of age. I was molested by a family friend's daughter, who was double my age. She told me not to tell my parents because it was our "special secret", that "this is the way people show their love for each other", for some reason in my brain I keep thinking "my parents would say I'm lying". I don't remember her telling me this word for word, but that is how I felt. So I kept quiet, never said a word. My parents and I moved to a different state, and somehow I put the abuse out of my mind. I actually "forgot" about it for several years. My memory of my early childhood from then until age 9 is more or less non-existent (I can remember bits and pieces). The first memory I really have, is of me cutting myself at the age of 9. At that time I didn't even know what I was doing had a name, all I knew is for some reason it made me feel better, so of course I kept doing it. I think somewhere in my 9 year old brain I knew it was abnormal, so I never told anyone, for fear it would be taken away from me. And everything at that point in my life felt so bad, I desperately wanted to feel better. I was teased in school for being the new kid, my dad was working all of the time, my mom was sick, and while she was "healthy" for someone with a chronic illness, I always had the fear of her dying looming over my head. And it was never talked about in our household. It was always about pretending that everything would be o.k. Additionally, we had moved thousands of miles away from all our family and friends. I remember feeling like I was alone, I felt really weird and abnormal. Things started getting worse at home, my dad took to drinking a lot, and he got really loud and angry a lot. My mom got really depressed. I felt the pressure to be perfect. I wanted to be perfect for my mom, so she didn't have to worry about me, I didn't want to be a burden, and I wanted to be perfect for my dad so he wouldn't yell at me and I wouldn't get in trouble. I just didn't feel good enough; I didn't feel like I measured up. Not in school with my peers, not for my teachers, not for my parents. I turned to food at the age of 12. For two years thereafter, I dabbled with compulsive eating. I remember one time in particular, I had gotten a ton of food in the school cafeteria, I was the odd-girl out, so I went into the girls bathroom, sat on the edge of the toilet, and crammed my face full of food. With each bite I compulsively ate, the bad feelings seeped out of me. That was my first experience with emotional eating. From that point on, I was hooked. Daily rituals of eating several portion sizes at every meal, PLUS snacks, and going to bed with a full tummy and completely numb, consumed my life. When I ate - I didn't feel. I liked that.

Unfortunately, compulsive eating came with a rather large price. Within two years (at the age of 14) I had piled on an ungodly amount of weight, and was now "FAT"! And not the "I think I'm fat, but really I'm not" type of fat, but the "I really am fat and my schoolmates and even the school nurse are shoving it in my face".

Things had gotten worse at home, and my parents decided to separate. My mom and I moved back to our hometown in New York, and my dad stayed in Texas. For the first time since I could remember I was truly happy. I was back in school with friends I went to Elementary school with, now several years later as teenagers. I felt loved and accepted for who I was. I even made the cheerleading squad! Life was good... Although I really did miss my dad. I was happy being back "home". Any "disordered eating" I had gone through had stopped completely. And so had the self injury. I was a normal, happy 14 year old.

By the end of my freshman year in high school my parents decided to give their marriage another try. So that meant leaving and saying good-bye to everyone, *AGAIN* and moving back to Texas. I felt like my world was ending. ALL I did was cry. My circle of friends threw me an awesome going away party, and I cried and cried and cried. The empty feeling came back. I became depressed, and considered suicide.

When we arrived back in Texas, things were o.k. for a while.. I got accepted to a "magnet school" for my sophomore year of high school. Only a handful of people were accepted into each school year at a time. My parents were *SO* proud. At this point my drive for perfection started coming back. I excelled in school to the max. I made National Honor Society, I was in Masterminds, I was in Honor's Classes. The sophomore class was only a class of just under 60 people. I knew pretty much everyone. And everyone knew me.

My life seemingly looked like I had it together. This is when I decided that I was going to lose weight, and nothing was going to get in my way! That way *everything* would really be perfect. That way *I* could really be perfect. So one of my best friends and I went on a "diet". I had tried diets countless times before and always "failed", and then was always ridiculed by my father for being fat, given suggestions by my mother on how to eat healthily. Their hearts were in the right place, my own mind was not. From there, my battle with Anorexia began. My friend quickly went off of her "diet", but I stumbled upon what - at that time - considered being the best thing in the entire world. I could live on virtually no food, I could exercise for a really long time, and the weight fell off, and quickly. Voila, problem solved right? Wrong. Within two years I had gone from "the fat girl" to "the really sick emaciated girl". Eventually, I became weak. My hair was falling out. My teeth started getting transparent. My skin was this yellow-ish grey color. I had really dark circles under my eyes. And I had really foul breath (which is common with Anorexic's). It hurt to sit down. But it hurt to stand too. I was NEVER comfortable and I was ALWAYS cold. But I never showed any of it, not even to myself. I'd always deny any of these things were real, or I'd make excuses and justifications. I started using amphetamines & marijuana, and went from being a casual smoker to smoking about a pack a day. At this point, I started cutting myself again. I felt so out of control, but I kept saying to myself "If you starve, you are IN control. If you eat you are weak and out of control". But I knew, logically I knew, I was out of control. I just wouldn't let myself (or anyone else) believe it. My parents put me in therapy, which really was pretty useless at that time, because I was in such denial, I had no desire to get better, and I lied about everything. My parents would get angry at me and frustrated with me. They'd tell me I was just trying to get attention and that I was being selfish and self centered. Of course, I already felt worthless enough, and them saying this just made me feel worse.

It only got worse from there. My parents divorced when I was 16 years old. My mom and I moved here to Houston.

My days and nights kind of just ran into one, it was all just one really long day -- I was completely obsessed. It was almost a game. How little can I eat today? How much can I lose today? How long can I exercise today? One day, when I was

16 years old, I came home from school. I was walking behind a friend of mine, and she climbed up on the ledge to get to the gate to our apartment complex. I'd say the ledge was only about 4 feet tall. Well I couldn't climb up on the ledge. I was too weak, I felt as though my legs were jello, I literally just wanted to lay down on the pavement and go to sleep. I walked through the apartment door, with a fake smile plastered on my face, and my mom said "I saw you through the window; you couldn't even get up on that itty bitty ledge, Jess... You're sick and you need help". I didn't know this then, but my mom told me when I was in treatment the 1st time, that she used to check on me several times in the middle of the night to make sure I was still breathing.

Of course, I thought she was out of her mind! I wasn't nearly thin enough yet, or perfect enough yet. I kept saying to myself "When I'm thin enough, then I'll start eating". Thing was, I never was thin enough. Ever. My "goal weights" kept getting lower and lower and lower. I would always ask people that I thought were skinny how much they weighed, if it was less than what I weighed, then that would be my goal weight. But when I got to that weight, I always felt and saw just as much fat, if not more, as before. So then I'd decrease my goal weight. Until it went lower and lower and lower. It was NEVER good enough, I NEVER felt good enough. I NEVER felt thin enough, or pure enough, or in control enough. But I was totally convinced that when I hit the perfect number on the scale, then I finally would feel on top of the world.

I will never forget that one day a group of girls came up to me at school and asked me if I had Cancer, to this day, 10 years later, I remember what I was wearing on that particular day. I was wearing my favorite outfit - the one that made me look the thinnest! Ironically enough the same night my mom said to me while we were in the grocery store, with a really disturbed look on her face that I looked like I was dying of cancer.

Another night I was working out at the gym, and I went into the Sauna. Next thing I knew I woke up in the Sauna, drenched with sweat and very dehydrated my heart beating really funny. I had passed out in the sauna, and to this day I have no idea how long I was passed out for. I never told anyone that.

Any healthy person would obviously see this was pure insanity!! But not me, really I had a rhyme and reason and justification for everything. I had convinced myself that really nothing was that bad...

I got into a very abusive relationship around this time, long story short, I was repeatedly raped and more or less brainwashed. He was very controlling, and my parents warned me against him. I cannot tell you how many fights my parents and I had about this boyfriend! I was angry at my parents, I actually screamed at my mom "I HATE YOU!!", to this day I still feel bad for that !! But being the stubborn 16 year old I was, I thought I was in love. And I thought surely he'd love me too, if only I was "better" than what I was. If I was "perfect" then he wouldn't treat me the way he did. Or maybe I deserved to be treated that way? Surely this was something that I could "fix". It never occurred to me to break off the relationship! This is when I turned to bulimia. I had NEVER made myself throw up before. The very thought of even putting food in my body disgusted me, and I really really hated throwing up. When I was younger and I would throw up if I got sick or something, I would get into crying fits and get a lot of anxiety.

I remember the very first time I purged. One of the very few things I would eat was this one particular Chinese restaurant, on the other side of town. So my mom would make the drive and we'd go eat together, God my poor mother. The things I put that woman through (throwing plates of food at her head, for one, screaming at her, causing such worry, etc.) On one particular day, I decided I wanted to go eat (which was like a hallmark-moment in our house), so my mom took me to the Chinese restaurant. Normally, I just pushed the food around on my plate, nibbled here and there, but never really consumed all that much. But this day was different. I finished several full plates of food. I am sure my mom was shocked! I hadn't finished an entire meal in years. Of course I became panic stricken, so I went into the bathroom with the intent of purging, but the bathroom was really crowded, and I just couldn't bring myself to do it around other people. I knew what I had to do, even if I had to wait until I got home to do it, the food WAS coming out of me.

And so the drive home was excruciating. The anxiety, the fear, the panic, the silent tears.... I about wanted to crawl out of my skin.

What is normally a 25 minute car ride, seemed like days.

Finally we got home.

And I purged for the first time.

That's when the bargaining began "Ok, I will only do this in desperate situations... Only when absolutely necessary".

But over a short period of time, the frequency of my binge/purge episodes drastically increased, going from maybe once every two weeks, to several times a day. Anorexia was now a memory, and Bulimia was my life...

I changed therapists at this point, to an eating disorders specialist, because I had no good luck with any of my previous therapists. I don't know if that was because of my lack of willingness, or their ignorance.

In 1998 I went off to college... I stopped binging and purging, and started starving myself again. Not only was I swimming several hours a day, but I was at the gym all of the time. At school I had free reign to do whatever my little heart desired and no one could stop me! So I ran with the "opportunity". I started using amphetamines again. And drinking quite a bit. I had dropped some weight, the cutting was out of control, and I began exhibiting symptoms of mental illness. Just short of the 1st semester, I had a nervous breakdown, called my mom to come pick me up, and left college.

I moved in with my new boyfriend, and the eating disorder, self injury, and mental illness symptoms continued. At this point I had upped the stakes to daily laxative, diet pill, and diuretic abuse.

Within a year I wound up in the E.R. with rectal hemorrhaging.

I started going to Texas Children's Hospital to see a doctor that specialized in eating disorders. Man, I hated that woman!! She saw RIGHT threw me, she called me on ALL my lies, she was really strict, and told me how it was. While part of me wanted to hate her, I also knew she could really help me, and for that I respected her. And I really did want help. I got put on a Halter Monitor (it's like a portable EKG machine that you have to wear strapped to you, and then you return it to the doctors, and the doctors review the results to see what your heart patterns are like - normal or abnormal) Six months passed, before my treatment team determined I had to go inpatient. I was 20 years old.

I spent 7 weeks at a treatment center in Florida, and had a very positive experience there. The staff was wonderful, the women I was there with and I became very close. But it was A LOT of hard work, very tiring, and so hard facing all the things that I had run from since childhood. I had been on psychiatric meds for a while at this point, but they changed all my meds while I was there, and did a complete psychiatric work up on me.

I left the treatment center shortly before Halloween of 2000.

And this is where my "affair" with relapse begins.

For the first year after I got out of treatment, I did extremely well. I had my "slips" behavior wise, but was more so on the up and up. My thought patterns though, had quickly reverted back to the way I had thought before I went to treatment. The worthlessness, the anxiety, the fear, the need for perfection, wanting to numb out, etc. I don't remember how or when I relapsed for the first time. When I say relapse, I want to make it clear that there is a difference between a "relapse" and a "lapse". A relapse is when you stay stuck in eating disorder behavior, when you are so obsessed you lose touch of reality. A "lapse" is a normal part of recovery, you fall - you get up - you brush yourself off - you try again.

From the year 2002-2005 I went to another residential treatment facility for a week long eating disorder intensive program, did an IOP program for five and a half months, and was in the psychiatric hospital for my eating disorder and self injury on 3 different occasions. Not to mention in therapy, therapy, therapy, I had begun seeing a dietician once a week, and started seeing a new psychiatrist once a month. During this time period I had been on just about every psychiatric medication out there, on heavy doses of them, and at one point I was up to 7 different kinds every day! I became addicted to one of my medications, abusing it as a way to not feel. It made me numb. At this point I was in such pain, I needed to be numb. One evening, I intentionally overdosed. I was fed up, done, through. I couldn't live the way I was living anymore. I was in too much pain, and I was causing too much pain. Within about three to five minutes after taking the pills, I came to my senses of what I had just done, realized I really did not want to die, freaked out, and purged up all the pills.

I had already somehow miraculously defeated death on more then one occasion. I remember going to bed every night (when I'd actually allow myself sleep) and I prayed and prayed and prayed to a higher-being (if there was one) to please please spare my life, if my life was spared, I would never act out on my eating disorder again. And my life was spared, for years and years; I woke up every day, only to start the cycle all over again. I also had programmed 9-1-1 into my portable phone, and every time I went to purge, I would take the phone with me into the bathroom and have it set to dial just incase something happened and I had a heart attack, or purged too much blood, or something else catastrophic.

My last couple of psychiatric stays did something to me. I had gone to the E.R. and needed stitches because of self injury, and was transported VIA ambulance to the psych hospital, which was some 30+ miles away, and this was just three days after I had been discharged from the same hospital! I was admitted to the Psych ICU (Intensive Care Unit) - which is where the very acute "cases" go. I looked around me - at the people I was with. Adults who were in their own world, some carrying baby dolls (my roommate, actually!! I actually found it quite comical, because I had seen the movie "Girl Interrupted", and a character in that movie is holding a baby doll. I surely thought "omg I really AM crazy!!), some smelling of a mixture of body odor, feces and cigarette smoke, others talking out loud to themselves. I was actually the most "normal" one on the unit - but I was put on that unit for precaution measures, and assured they would transfer me to the "adult unit" when they knew I was stable enough. My first night in the Psych ICU, I sat in my bed and cried and cried and cried. I DID NOT BELONG THERE! It was sooooooo depressing!!! And it was sad because the children's unit was upstairs above the ICU - and I could hear the children yelling and it made me so sad, some of them as young as 6 years old!!

Thankfully, within four days I was transferred to the adult unit, which actually was rather nice, I made some friends, and it was pretty "normal" up there. I was finally allowed to go to the cafeteria and eat meals down there (where as in the ICU I had to eat on the unit and was not allowed near a bathroom for an hour after I ate b/c my first stay at the psych hospital I purged my way through the entire stay!) Anyways, on the adult unit we had very interesting conversations on the smoke porch, the staff was pretty cool. I stayed for an additional week and a half.

I got out of the hospital the day before Thanksgiving 2005...

My therapist whom I had been seeing since 1998 had told me that she was no longer going to be seeing clients on an individual basis, and she was just going to be running the IOP program (and I was not in the program at that time), so she would not be able to see me anymore. She also said that even if that wasn't the case, she would most likely of referred me to somebody else. I was so upset! I had been seeing her since 1998!! I looked up to her and admired her. I felt like a really big failure at this point, because she said she would have referred me out, in my mind meaning that I was a) untreatable b) I let her down. This was one of the most admirable women I had ever met. She never gave up hope that I would recover. She believed in me, when very very few people did. I truly believe had it not been for her, I would have given up. Stopping therapy with her was one of the hardest things I have had to do in my life. She will forever hold a special place in my heart. It is now, in hindsight, that I see that everything really does happen for a reason, and while we may not like it - or agree with it - at the time, eventually we see the meaning behind everything.

I started seeing a new therapist, an eating disorders specialist who I had a history with b/c I went to her support group on and off for several years, so I already felt comfortable with her, and she knew some of my history. One of my best friend's also sees this therapist, and she has a lot of experience and good results. So there was no doubt in my mind that I wanted to start seeing her. I continued seeing my dietician and psychiatrist as well.

I started seeing a great deal of improvement almost immediately. My thinking began to change, I became able to cry again, the only time I had really ever cried in years was when I was at the hospital. My eating disorder behaviors drastically decreased, the cutting stopped completely. I began seeing the world "in color" rather than in "black and white". The glass went from half empty to half full. I don't know, it's weird. It's almost like one day I just had this "awakening", and I knew everything was going to be just fine. I knew I was going to be o.k. It happened, just like that..... I don't know why it happened when it did, and at this point I don't much care. I am just grateful it did. I try not to analyze or judge but just accept and use the knowledge I have gained towards a positive attitude and healthy and balanced lifestyle.

Recovery from my eating disorder, strong solid recovery, was made up of a lot of ups and downs. A lot of feelings and emotions, sometimes I felt like I was just going to explode. I still lived in a lot of fear and doubt. Doubt that I could ever fully recover; fear that I would fail once again. I was TERRIFIED about stepping into the unknown, into unfamiliar territory. But what it came down to for me was this: The risk it would be to get into and stick with recovery was FAR LESS then the risk I would be taking staying sick, risking my sanity, and eventually the inevitable: death. I had already had 2 friends of mine die from their eating disorders (and one was at a "normal" weight!! You can DIE from an eating disorder at ANY weight!! Eating disorders are NOT about the number on the scale)

Today, life is good. I am HAPPY (yes, I still have my bad days though!), I have peace and serenity today. I have an identity today. I have a social life. I know how to genuinely smile and laugh and *FEEL* I don't have that blank lifeless look in my eyes, my eyes glow... I eat "normally", I never think about the eating disorder or self injury - and if ever I do think about it it's more like I think about the fact that I don't think about it! I am down to just an anti-depressant every day, and then an anti-psychotic PRN (as needed).

Today I consider myself recovered. It's such a wild feeling. It feels like a huge accomplishment, it has totally put a different perspective on the way I perceive and process things. While I often wonder what my life would have been like had I not developed an eating disorder or became a cutter, and while I wish more than anything that I could have spared myself and my parents the pain we all went through during my many years being sick, I have to say I have no regrets. Going through what I have been through, has shaped who I am as a person today. I truly believe I am a more authentic, more genuine, more accepting, and more insightful person because of my struggles and latter journey through recovery. Today I take *NOTHING* for granted. From the smallest things like my mom's puppy chasing a butterfly outside, to the biggest things.

Complete recovery IS possible, and it DOES happen. It can happen for ALL of those who suffer from an eating disorder. We are all beautiful people - both inside and out - and we should NOT let ANYONE (including the eating disorder) try to brainwash us into thinking any differently!!

I think the biggest lessons I have learned in my recovery have been this:

* There is no such thing as perfection. It simply does not exist. It's an illusion we create in our minds. The more we strive for perfection, the less we find it,

the more we hate ourselves, and think we're just not being "good enough", and this perpetuates the self destructive cycle.

* Life really IS greener on "this" (recovery) side!!

* There is no such thing as failure, as long as you are trying (really truly trying!)

* Perseverance pays off!!!!

* Use tools of recovery; they'll save your butt!!!

* And lastly, one of the biggest lessons I have learned in my own recovery has been that I had the power to recover *WITHIN* me, this entire time.... I just wasn't looking in the right place!! If I had used even half of the energy on recovery that I expended on maintaining my self destruction, I would have recovered YEARS ago!!!

By Jessica, 26. Houston, Texas USA. Suffered from COE (Compulsive Overeating) turned Anorexia turned Bulimia turned EDNOS (Eating Disorder Not Otherwise Specified) - total of 12 and a half years. 7 time Relapse-Survivor (from the year 2000 to 2005). Finally Fully Recovered! Childhood Sexual Abuse and Rape Survivor. Recovered Cutter. Diagnosed with Mental Illness. Symptom Free from Mental Illness for 1 year! If you want to get in touch with Jessica, please send an e-mail to ribbons_undone@sbcglobal.net.

Getting the Help You Need

By Kate Holden, 20. London, England. Anorexia from age 13. Self-Harm. Recovered. Teaching Assistant and part-time photography student, starting Midwifery degree in September 2006.

After a holiday in Crete, where I had already started experimenting with under eating, I remember distinctly the summer barbecue at a neighbour's had me in fits of tears about my weight; this was the day I decided to starve my body into submission.

I was the oldest child, very academic, and came into puberty at ten or eleven. Being the sort of child who liked to please her parents, I was terrified my body wasn't something I could readily control, and that womanhood brought the anxieties and depressions that I saw my mother struggling with. Through the last year of primary and the first year of secondary school I was tormented by close friends about being more 'grown up' than them and had the feeling of being sorely conspicuous amongst my peer group; I guess that the consistent build up of negative reactions to my maturing body triggered the drastic measures I took to remain in a child's guise.

Even when I had lost a considerable amount of weight, and my parents especially were commenting on how thin I looked, the drive to lose more didn't subside. In all ways I had retreated into myself, become completely closed off socially and emotionally, and intensely obsessed with what was measurable in my life: calories and kilos lost. I lived in a sort of coma, full of white noise, without feeling anything but fear. I was so afraid to stop or be stopped because I believed there was nothing outside of my bubble; bursting my impenetrable pupa would kill me - thrust out in a world where time would undo me. I could see the pain of others around me (my brothers too waiting in dread of what I might do next) but felt there was nothing I could do to relieve them of their guilt and worry and panic; I thought that the root of it all was outside of me, was something out of my control. Getting me out of my 'vacuum' and into a hospital was a lot of trouble for my parents, who pleaded for advice from various health professionals for many weeks before I was finally assessed by one of my mum's colleagues. I was admitted the same day, needless to say, because I was in such a bad state physically. Much of the initial information gathered about my condition at the time has been relayed to me; I was only really aware of feeling relieved at not having to think about my schoolwork, and the rows at home, which had been increasing as my weight fell.

I was glad too for my parents, who now wouldn't have to worry that their fourteen year old was starving, but instead being fed and monitored and counseled, as you would expect any child with a life-threatening disorder to be treated. Alas, it was a different story in reality! I was weighed every few days, but in between it was entirely up to me whether to eat, or exercise, or cheat my weight, or cut myself - the 'care' I received from that first hospital could be packaged and wrapped up in a box labeled 'Minimal intervention - miscellaneous condition - do not treat because we don't know how'!

One day I would be hooked up to a monitor telling them my heart rate was worryingly low, and that actually I might slip into a coma tonight, and the next without any further tests I could be doing a bit of frantic pacing after no breakfast or lunch, and chatting to the nurses about not really 'fancying' dinner without raising any real concern. I was once seen by the local child psychiatrist with my parents present, was thoroughly humiliated by his demeaning and inappropriate questions, burst into tears through the part when he insisted that a Section was my parents' best option, and can't really remember anything else he said - he treated me like I was possessed, and wouldn't it be nicer for everyone if I was contained in a proper little unit where they would know how to 'deal' with me. It was clear that the hospital was not equipped for helping patients with psychiatric conditions, but once they had admitted me, their medical intervention was elementary.

Luckily my mum is a pediatric nurse, had some connections at a different hospital, and we escaped with my things, pretending to go to the hospital shop, whilst my dad distracted the nurses. This was about the time I realised the incompetence of the professionals around me and the journey through various other hospitals and specialist units became a game, trying to convince them I was well and gaining weight - that they should let me go - and this was not uncommon, for the girls to pull the wool over the nurses' eyes in a collective effort to outwit the system. I became a very good anorexic during my inpatient treatment. I had no intention of putting on any significant amount of weight and in fact had quite a good time devising ways to hide food, finding ways to cheat at weigh-in, exercising vigorously between 'checks' and banging a drum in therapy sessions to relieve the abstract anger they were at pains to point out. No one addressed the disorder with any passion or hope for recovery - a senior nurse snidely remarked that she'd see me again in a few months time, after I'd relapsed - and the general consensus was that to get any sense out of an anorexic you'd have to wait until you'd fed her back to a normal weight. Force feeding via a nasogastric tube was often used, bulimic patients had access to their private toilets too soon after meals, many nurses were untrained in eating disorders and let it go by them when we hid food, poured drinks away and kept glass bottles for self-harm. I'm sure that most of them thought we should 'just eat'. I was amused by the therapy offered me, with its talk of 'managing' the disorder - I wanted to live as an anorexic or get out completely.

My day-patient care after leaving the specialist unit was dire. I was alone when eating, and my therapy sessions were ways of passing time until I left in the evening. I really didn't have much trust in improving my situation in the long term, after transferring to outpatient care at a different hospital, because my consultant treated anorexia as a biological demon that couldn't be exorcised. My weight dropped and my confusion rose - three months after leaving a five month inpatient treatment I was at a lower weight than when I had been admitted. I think a lot of people were ready to put me back into hospital and I have to say that their resignation to my illness did not instill a belief that I could escape it. But even as I sat in a room with my mother and my consultant, talking into his dictaphone about my deterioration like I was just a naughty little girl, I felt I knew from my session with Bob* (whom I had seen once before I went into that first hospital) that anorexia didn't have to be chronic.

I had been tricking them all for a chance to get out of hospital and try and see Dr. Bob on a regular basis - I started doing this I think the winter after I turned fifteen, with great success and a sense of independence, traveling between London and York on my own, proving the skeptical consultant wrong. I began to see that I wasn't a stupid and insolent child with an incurable disease but an adult with a fear of surviving without her parents.

By Kate Holden, 20. London, England. Anorexia from age 13. Self-Harm. Recovered. Teaching Assistant and part-time photography student, starting Midwifery degree in September 2006.

---

* Dr. Bob Johnson, Consultant Psychiatrist, England. Founder of The James Nayler Foundation. For more information, please go to **www.TruthTrustConsent.com**.

01/00

The first poem about my illness I wrote when I'd just turned 14 and was in hospital - it was kind of an opening up, an invitation to the people whom I needed to help me out of my hole.

Let me in
Let me see what you see
Let me think what you think
Show me the way, light my path
I'll do anything if you let me in
To your secret world
Where are you?
I'm searching
My eyes can still look
Even though my mind doesn't think
If you protect me now,
I'll protect you in years to come.
If you remember me now,
I'll never let you fade.
Don't let me waste my life - jump
in, come on inside,
I'll let you in.

By Kate Holden, 20. London, England. Anorexia from age 13. Self-Harm. Recovered. Teaching Assistant and part-time photography student, starting Midwifery degree in September 2006.

1/9/00

I wrote this to a friend who was finding it really hard to overcome her problems when we were in hospital together.

Michelle,
Knowing you as little as I do,
You can be sure, I'll remember you.
The mask that you wear,
That your body's locked in,
It is not steel,
Tis only tin.
You can get out, you will break free,
I only hope one day you'll see.

By Kate Holden, 20. London, England. Anorexia from age 13. Self-Harm. Recovered. Teaching Assistant and part-time photography student, starting Midwifery degree in September 2006.

31/1/01

*This poem I dedicated to my consultant when I left out patient treatment
– she helped me see things and believe in myself and my recovery.*

I flick through the pages that
Were once my life,
So dark then,
So full of light now.
Each page I turn
Tells another story of guilt,
How I couldn't let go –
Only punished the child I
was becoming,
The child I was.
And how things have changed,
Transformed,
I am no longer hidden from life,
I can never be so alone
Such as I was,
Tomorrow no longer brings
The hell it used to.
I can only ask the world,
Do not judge me from my past,
Take me as I come,
For this is me.

By Kate Holden, 20. London, England. Anorexia from age 13. Self-Harm.
Recovered. Teaching Assistant and part-time photography student, starting
Midwifery degree in September 2006.

My Eating Disorder Story

By Kim Ratcliffe, 44. British Columbia, Canada. Anorexia on and off for over 20 years. 12 years Recovery.

My name is Kim Ratcliffe, I am 44 years old, married (2nd marriage) to a wonderful man who loves "me" for me & not my body size! I have 3 children aged 17, 13, & 14. I have been recovering from anorexia for the past 12 years & had my eating disorder on and off for 20 years. I live in British Columbia, Canada.

My eating disorder began when I was about 15 or 16, but at that time, I did not know, that was what I had. I just thought it was the "norm". I rarely ate breakfast, and lunch was small, but I did eat dinner. I remember always watching what I ate, although I was never over weight. But for me, the one thing I had was my thinness. I always thought my thinness would bring me happiness, love and friends. I realize now, how wrong I have been. At the time, the other teenagers I knew were always in "awe" of me, because I was so thin. Little did they know how much I did not like who I was and that I starved myself. I remember one instance that stands out in my mind. It was my graduation year and I had a bet with another girl on "who would weigh the least." Unfortunately, I won, but at the time I felt so good about it, I was proud of what I had accomplished. I was married young so things pretty much stayed the same as far as eating, I would watch what I ate, but also treated myself. I did go to several exercise classes a week, to lose weight, but keep in mind I was never over weight. The only time I really ate, without thinking about it, so-to-speak, was when I was pregnant, but, I ate for the baby, not me!

Now we come to the time when my anorexia became very present. It was March 1994, I was 34 years old, and it was on my oldest son's 5th birthday. I woke up that morning, looked at myself in the mirror, and said "I am fat. It's time to go on a diet." There were so many things that were out of control at this time! I had to have a hysterectomy, (I wanted more children) but I didn't want one, my (then husband) lost his job and overall just felt stressed to the max. However I knew I could lose weight, I had the power and something I had control over. No one could make me eat. I had a goal weight set in my mind (I was never over weight). I did succeed in getting there. I began using a diet drink. I would have that for breakfast, a light lunch and dinner. I did this for a few months. Then I just began drinking coffee for most of my day, but I would eat some dinner. As time went on all I would have is coffee, and small quantities of other foods, allowing myself only a certain amount of calories a day or less. I would weigh myself several times a day. By August of that year, I found out that my family physician was moving to relocate. I was crushed!! I had heard that there was usually something that throws you over to the "other side" so-to-speak, and this was it for me. We had a nice relationship. You also just don't wake up one morning and say "gee I think I will become anorexic". I started out in control of my eating but by now the eating disorder had control over me!!! I decided if I lost more weight and became sicker he would stay, I was wrong of course, he still left. When I was in therapy I realized what his relationship meant to me and how I took it. In my opinion, everyone has deep, core issues, because **FOOD is NOT THE ISSUE**, my big issue was abandonment, as I discovered in therapy. About this time I began using the laxatives.. My weight became lower and lower. Friends began to comment on how good I looked, which I enjoyed hearing. However, they didn't know what was going on with me. It starts out as a huge secret (or it did for me) but in the end the secret is revealed.

I was now introduced to the new doctor taking over. I had quite the attitude with her. She informed me that she would only be there a week and then was off for a month due to a prior commitment. So, I left the office and said to the receptionist (who at the time was the only person I felt safe talking to) "I will be a certain weight" when she gets back." We are now in October and true to my words that is what I weighed when she got back. By now I had no interest in friends, I wasn't sleeping, and I was cold all the time, exhausted beyond belief, of course not eating and now having heart pains. I always cared for my children; they were always fed very well, just not me.

It was about 2 weeks before my new doctor was due back and I call it my "bottom out" period. I was still using laxatives, but this time, I could not make it to the bathroom and I went everywhere. I was so ashamed and felt so guilty. I called up the receptionist and said "I think I need help." By now most of my friends and my (then husband) thought I was anorexic, told me so, but I didn't believe them until that moment when I spoke with the receptionist. I was soooooooooo tired of hearing the voices in my head saying "don't eat this, don't eat that, if you do eat, you MUST get rid of it, the more weight you lose the happier you will be, I am your only friend." I was tired of fighting and I wanted out. When the doctor got back I went to see her and said "I need help." That night I told my (then husband) what was happening and that I would be going into the hospital the next day, I did.

I was scared to death of what would happen to me, but never realizing till much later how sick I really was. I remember drinking those little juices, and crying for 10 minutes. I felt so ashamed and so guilty, I was a bad person. I was there for 9 days. In November I had an assessment with the eating disorder doctor there. To this day I still remember him asking me to push my hands and feet against him and him saying "at 34 you have the muscle tone of a 9 year old." It still freaks me out when I see this, not realizing how ill I really was.

In January 1995 I went into the in-patient program at St. Paul's Hospitals eating disorder program for adults. I was there for 3 weeks and I learned a lot about myself and my eating disorder. It was a difficult time there. But it wasn't until April of 1995 that I decided to do there 3 month out-patient program. This gave me my "quick start" as I like to call it, on how to not only learn to eat again, but of course looking more into my issues and learning "new tools" on how to handle my anorexia. When I left there I felt so good and so much more in control. It was there that I met a wonderful woman, a nurse clinician named Linda Lauritzen, within the eating disorder program. She was the one I began to trust and knew about my abandonment issues and promised to help me through them. I was also introduced to my therapist, whom I saw for 5 years, Lynn Redenbach. Both of these women I credit to my recovery. They were both there, to support me and work with me and never gave up on me!!

After the out patient program I was up and down for about 2 years, then one day I had a major break through again. I was in Linda's office very anorexic and I said to her "why can't you just accept me the way I am, anorexic." She said she would never do that, that she would be there for me, support me but would never support anorexia. I began crying and could feel myself come out and the anorexia leaving. I believe I was so afraid of losing Linda in my life (remember I have abandonment issues) that I finally "heard" what she was saying and everyone else around me. It was from this point on (1997) that I have never looked back. I began eating my meals, gaining weight, yes freaking out about it, but dealing with it in therapy. I was able to discover the issues that needed to be looked at, deal with them, and find out who I was and in time learn to love myself.

To this day, I am still doing great. Do I have bad and good days, of course I do, I am human. But I also know that when I am having a bad day, it's a red flag for me to look at what is going on around me, what could be bothering me. These days do not happen often anymore!!!

I have finally learned to love me, that I am a good person, that I don't need to be thin in order to be loved (which is what I thought), that I do deserve to be loved and can love back. This is the happiest I have ever been in my life. I have learned that the number on the scale means nothing (by the way I do not own a scale), its what is inside that counts. There are days I still have body image issues, but I am able to work through them. My now husband, Tom, is wonderful and very supportive. He has helped me understand relationships better, communicate more, not being afraid to feel or say what I feel, and knowing that I can rely on myself for my needs. My abandonment issues are next to gone now as I am able to depend on myself. I will never go back to where I was, I have worked too hard for where I am today to give that back to my anorexia. And in a strange way now, I see my eating disorder differently, not as an enemy, not necessarily as a friend, but as something that has brought me to where I am today, because if I had not gone through what I did, I would not have learned about myself and grown as a person, and for that I am thankful.

My life is good now, fulfilled. I don't count calories or fat. I eat what I want when I want. I have learned that in order to do the things I love in life, whether that be work or my hobby's or walking or just spending time with my family, what ever it is, that I have to eat. I have to give my body "fuel", and that is with food. When I feed my body, in return it gives me the energy to do the things I love. **This is the happiest I have ever been in my life and how ironic the most I have ever weighed.**

Don't ever give up the fight to recover. It is possible to be in recovery, yes it takes a lot of hard work, determination, strength you name it, but it is so worth it. **Living without anorexia controlling my life is such a wonderful feeling, and an even better feeling, knowing I have control of my life!!"**

By Kim Ratcliffe, 44. British Columbia, Canada. Anorexia on and off for over 20 years. 12 years Recovery. For more information on Kim's personal journey and her journal writings, go to **http://www.angelfire.com/oh3/anorexia** or send an email to **kvrat@shaw.ca.**

Scars from a Recovered Life

By Izayana, 23. Mexico. Anorexia for 12 years. Depression. Self-Harm. Recovered.

Hi, my name is Izayana, I'm Mexican. I'm a psychologist, specialized in teenagers and group therapy. I'm also an English teacher in junior high and an art teacher in elementary school, and run my own business, a gift shop, study artistic photography, and specialize in Neurolinguistic-Programming. But all these things are not the reason that brings me here today, to share my story... My name is Izayana, I'm 23 years old, and I'm a former anorexic. My anorexia started when I was eleven years old and it has been a long road for me.

It started suddenly, I wasn't really fat, or I never thought about it. It was never a big deal for me, my looks or appearance. I had a very hard childhood, but I made myself strong because I had to be. You know this obsession that most anorexic girls have, "the perfect girl syndrome". I forced myself for so long that I just fell apart, I never knew what was the first thing, or if one thing lead to the other, but by the time I turned 12, I had anorexia and a huge depression. Back then in my town we hadn't heard a lot about it and it wasn't "hip" like it is now, so it wasn't a fashion thing like they said. It just was my only way to deal with problems. My psychologist told me once that I "ate" all my feelings, thoughts and tears for so long that there wasn't any space for food... I was very young then but I just quit eating, it was great because I finally had control over something. The only thing I didn't see was that the anorexia controlled me. I didn't know I had this problem, and they just thought that was a teen thing. They focused on my depression, and the huge change I made, of being a bright, sparkly, funny, easy going happy little girl. In 24 hours I was this bittered, always sad, blue, antisocial adolescent. The rollercoaster began... I kept myself into the limits, and I got periods where I ate normally and then went back to my eating disorder - and my weight dropped.

I realize now that it was the only way I found to punish myself, to finish with the life I hated so badly. I tried to kill myself so many many times... I was a cutter too, anything that could make me feel bad, was ok for me. I passed out several times, and had anemia, but it was such a way of life that I had never thought that there was any other way. I went to many doctors, psychologists, and psychiatrics, but when I was 17 I had a "sabbatical year" from my disease. I was doing alright, also with depression, the fights with my mom ended, everything stopped... for a while. I entered college, I chose psychology (hahaha) I wondered why?, but the good days were over. I began losing a lot of weight and reached my lowest weight ever and my hair started to fall out. I passed out every single day; I could spend a couple of days in a row without any food. I took many diet pills, and I had a little notebook where I wrote down every single thing I ate and how many calories it had. I did a couple of hours of exercise at night so I didn't sleep. I hid myself every time I got sick; thinking about it right now makes me cry. It was so amazingly insane; I was entering hospitals every week. I got osteoporosis, early menopause, liver disease, kidney disease, heart disease.... I was dying, my wishes were coming true. I got 15 days in the hospital for parenteral nutrition. Three months later I had to have a gastrostomic procedure done. I had a tube inserted in my stomach where they fed me, and I still would find ways to get rid of the food. All this right now seems to me so far away, but still so close, so real. It was me who did that, not a movie actress or a model, no! A normal person, a family girl, a straight A's student, me!! All those insane actions; all those Hollywood movie moments I lived them; all that damage to myself; was me the one that did it; the one that today stands in front of a classroom full of kids; or a crowd of people to listen to a conference; the one that despite of all that is still alive. Finally I entered therapy, and started the long, hard road of recovery. Of course it was hard. Of course it hurt. I entered a rehab clinic (Oceanica in Mexico), where I spent 3 months, 3 long months where I had to fight against a way of life I was used to. The principal form the clinic told me once, 'I believe in you, there's a reason you survived all that, thanks for existing!' Those were the most beautiful heart-breaking words that I heard back then. Me? I deserve to live, and live - not only survive?, to cry and laugh and feel? After that, once I was out I had to continue by myself. I went back to the thing I knew but I realized that I can do it, that it was up to me and that no matter what happened I had and have continued fighting for my life, no one else is going to. I had some difficult experiences. I survived an assault and came out of it really injured. One month later, two car accidents, and some other things that showed me that I was on the recovery path but that life would go on and things would continue to happen whether I wanted it or not.

All this was 3 years ago... it has been hard, but in every way it has been different. I never ever thought I could live, not just survive. I have felt everything good or bad. I have been conscious about it, and the most important thing, I feel ALIVE.... everything is possible. I'm about to start studying a masters degree in addiction and eating disorder counseling. Service is my motor, and sharing my experience with other girls out there that are just like me, who think there is no way out of this, is for me the only reason I'm proud I had anorexia.

With all my love, I dedicate my recovery to all of you suffering form an eating disorder, because there is a way.

By Izayana, 23. Mexico. Anorexia for 12 years. Depression. Self-Harm. Recovered.

THE PAIN OF MY HEART

The pain I feel in my heart is very deep.
It never goes away even in my sleep.
Sometimes I want to cry, but at times I can not.
So when I feel like this, I just lie down and sigh.

I want the pain to go away.
And yet it seems it keeps me at bay.
I used to starve, binge, and purge.
Now I try to resist the urge.

But now I cut.
Therefore I feel like I'm stuck in a rut.
Always doing something to get rid of the pain
Yet I realize it's not much of a gain.

I don't know how to cope.
Yet I don't want to groan and mope.
So I try to alleviate the pain.
This in turn makes me feel like I'm going insane.

Someday the pain will end
Now I just try to mend.
Mend my broken heart
Until I can make a fresh start
And say goodbye to the pain, the pain of my heart.

By Whitney Laree Greenwood Johnson, 18. Multiethnic. Single. Social Service Student. Salem, Oregon, United States. Bulimic but went through an Anorexic stage, Excessive Dieter, for almost 8 years. In Recovery. Have Self Injured on occasion mostly recovered from that. Depression, Anxiety, Panic Disorder, Under Control. Recovered from Suicidal Thoughts, have attempted Suicide. Attention Deficit Hyperactivity Disorder.

DEAR ENEMY

You promised to be my friend, but a false friend you were.

I turned to you for self esteem, you lowered my self esteem.

I came to you for comfort, you only caused me torment.

I came to you when I was sad, you didn't make me happy.

I came to you to help me calm down when I was under stress, the relief was only temporary.

I came to you to feel accepted, you made me feel worthless.

I came to you to get respect from other people, it made no difference.

I tried to throw my burdens on you; you only gave more to carry on my shoulders.

I came to you to feel safe, you increased my fear.

I came to you for companionship, you made me lonelier.

I came to you to fill a void; you made me felt just as empty.

I loved you, cherished you, I fought to keep you.

I wouldn't let others take you away from me.

But even when I decided that I wanted you gone.

You wouldn't leave. You tried to hold me in your vice.

You still try to force your way into my life.

You will not win oh enemy of mine, I will fight you until the end.

Why can't you hear me I don't want you anymore?

Good By and Good By Forever.

Who is this enemy? An eating disorder.

By Whitney Laree Greenwood Johnson, 18. Multiethnic. Single. Social Service Student. Salem, Oregon, United States. Bulimic but went through an Anorexic stage, Excessive Dieter, for almost 8 years. In Recovery. Have Self Injured on occasion mostly recovered from that. Depression, Anxiety, Panic Disorder, Under Control. Recovered from Suicidal Thoughts, have attempted Suicide. Attention Deficit Hyperactivity Disorder.

A Revelation

By Katherine Roemer, 19. Kentucky, USA. 7 years with EDNOS (Eating Disorder Not Otherwise Specified) and Anorexia. Sexual Assault and Abuse Survivor. Self-Harm. Recently Declared Recovered.

They say to recover you need to have a life changing revelation.
I say you need to have two – one to begin recovery and one to finish it.

My first revelation came at the age of sixteen. I had spent the past four years in the grips of my eating disorder--the first three under Eating Disorder Not Otherwise Specified (EDNOS) and the last under full blown Anorexia Nervosa. By the time I had reached my low weight, my entire body would ache from the cold. Warm water and heating pads didn't help; the cold was coming from the inside. I was starving and anemic. Moving or thinking about anything besides my weight was difficult to do. I couldn't remember anything, anyway. Lying in a warm bathtub became my favorite past time, but it wasn't always a pleasant experience. I would cry every time I had to look down at my body. I closed my eyes and felt my back being bruised by my protruding spine against the bottom of the tub. It calmed me, but I couldn't get out without leaving behind a handful of hair--and that was before I brushed out the tangles. It wasn't until an emotional breakdown that I decided to make a change. I got tired of dying. I called a therapist instead.

The way an eating disorder works is like Obsessive Compulsive Disorder, a drug addiction, or any other problem, really. You perform some task so you don't have to deal with your inner emotions. To get rid of the problem you must stop the rituals and then learn how to live without them.

In the beginning, the rules are pretty simple. You eat. You show up at a meal, concentrate, try to eat as much as is on the plate, then secretly go back to your room and spend the next hour or so in the fetal position certain that you are about to die until the food has been slowly digested. That is how it goes for a while, at least until your stomach is able to hold more food at a time. You're definitely not recovered, though. You never stopped weighing. If you had it would mean that you would really be giving up your eating disorder, and that's something you just can't think about yet. One step at a time, right? Eventually it does get easier to eat a meal, look at yourself in the mirror, and not care about whether the scale is left out with no one else home--but the real problem still exists, and it has nothing to do with food.

I call it the "In-Between". It's that period of time where you're recovering but not recovered. It's when you really begin to feel out of control, but no one will help you because you're no longer on the verge of starving yourself to death. It's probably the longest part of recovery with the greatest risk of relapse, but it's also where I grew the most as a person.

Even as I was learning to love the body I was in, I still had difficulty learning to love the person I was on the inside. In the past, I had silently endured repeated sexual assault and emotional abuse from various sources, including the relationship I was in at the time. It was no wonder that I valued myself so little. There were many occasions where I would surrender to an anxiety attack or lash out in anger, sometimes becoming violent towards my significant other. Every other time I was content in being violent only to myself. Although I had already vowed to recover, at the age of seventeen I continued to battle my depression and insecurities with pill popping, self-injury, restricting my food intake, compulsive exercising, and compulsive overeating. I also spent many nights contemplating or attempting suicide. My second revelation would take place at a short term inpatient facility.

A year and a half ago I was in "recovery" and heading towards my low weight. I was also sitting in an evaluation room of a hospital, surrounded by doctors and nurses. They diagnosed me with "a little bit of anorexia," known to the non-medically retarded as EDNOS, along with Major Depression. I was given a week and a bottle of pills before they determined that I was stable. I took them for two weeks before adding the remainder to my collection of pills I was saving for an overdose.

Sometimes a revelation takes place in one night. Sometimes it has to develop over a period of time. If all we plan to do is wait for it, we might as well take steps to help speed up the process. Three weeks after my release I separated from my abusive relationship. Eight months after my release I threw away my razorblades and pills. Four months after that I threw them away again. How did I find the strength? The last year and a half has been spent drowning myself in therapy-based TV shows, movies, books, and websites. I began writing and continued to draw and sculpt. I shifted my focus towards college to study Psychology and Social Work. Revelations started to be found all over the place.

What I've learned is simple. Recovery stems from constant discovery. You have to take what you've learned and adapt. Take steps and risks that you would normally be afraid to. Mourn for what you've lost and celebrate what you've gained. Allow yourself to grow. Practice being happy, because for the unlucky 99% of us, it isn't going to come naturally. Part of that is learning how to forgive. Above all, know that recovery is going to take time. The most important lesson is that sometimes the mind just needs to figure a thing or two out on its own.

By Katherine Roemer, 19. Kentucky, USA. 7 years with EDNOS (Eating Disorder Not Otherwise Specified) and Anorexia. Sexual Assault and Abuse Survivor. Self-Harm. Recently declared recovered.

What Is the End for the Caterpillar, Is a New Beginning for the Butterfly

By Shinyflower, 23. Nurse. Norway. Anorexia for 6 years. Recovered.

I thought recovery was about gaining weight. I feared it as my worst enemy.

I now know that I was wrong. Recovery can on a physical level be about gaining the weight the body needs to do its job. It can be about learning to eat more and eat more often, but this doesn't have to be the main focus for recovery!

I found out that recovery is about learning to live, instead of just existing as a body. I learned that recovery is about finding a life that works for me, a life based on my talents, my dreams and my limits. It's about learning to live my life, not the life others have prepared for me. It's about accepting that I am not perfect and I will never be perfect. I have my limits, I have areas in my life that I am not good at. But I also learned that I don't have to be perfect. I am okay the way I am right here, right now. I don't have to change. I don't have to do something to be worthy of life. I don't have to do anything to deserve the love from others. I am okay the way I am… If others don't like me for who I am, then it's their problems, not mine. I can accept myself and choose to be with people that accept me for who I am.

I don't have to be a good girl all the time. I have the same rights as everybody else on earth. I have the right to take up the space my body takes. I don't have to make excuses for being alive and for breathing. I don't have to apologize for my thoughts and my feelings. I have the right to be me… I have the right to cry, scream, need things, be loved, love, be happy and be sad.

For me recovery was much about learning to accept me for who I am. Accept the body I have. Accept that I don't have the family I dreamed of. I can't make my family the perfect family by starving myself to something I thought was a perfect body…

My recovery started with a little act of kindness to myself every day. I started to say "I love you" to the reflection in the mirror, even though I didn't believe my own words. But nice words do something with you, and little by little I learned to love myself. I learned to take care of myself. I learned to like me and be good to me. It was not something that happened over one night. And it was not easy. It cost me a lot of tears, courage, strength and faith… There were times when I wanted to give up, but I learned that it was those times that it was most important for me to keep walking and also reach out to others for help.

The eating disorder has cost me a lot… I had to spend six awful years living with the ed, my physical body collapsed and I nearly died, I lost some of my friends, before I realized that I was playing with death and I had to choose what road I really wanted to take. One day I just realized that I had to choose life or death.

I chose life… And I am now considering myself recovered… Recovery is not only having good days, but it is handling those bad days in a healthy way. It's knowing that the sun will come up again.

Even though it has cost me a lot of hard work. Even though I gained some weight and have had to throw away some of my trousers. I believe recovery is worth its cost.

I am finally seeing the sunshine again. I live in colors. I have learned to feel again. For years I was numb. And if I felt anything it was pain. I am little by little learning to dance in the sunshine and smell the flowers along the road. And I have opened up my eyes to see the love that's in my life and always have been there, but I was too blinded by the eating disorder to see it… And I am starting to love myself again… I haven't had interest in and time for boys in years, but finally I am starting to enjoy that we were created man and female.

I have found a life that works for me. I have learned to speak with my body instead of with my weight. I have learned to talk about my needs instead of screaming my needs out with my starvation. I have learned to take time to rest and to take care of me. I have learned to listen to my body.

It feels like I have really moved into my body and made a home out of it. I've got the light in my eyes back and the smile on my face are finally real.

Finally I have energy enough for living.

I have time for life…

I feel alive…

Many people feel sorry for me, for wasting away six years of my youth on the ed, but I feel that I have been more lucky than many people… At a young age, I have learned to know myself. I know my limits and I know what I am made of. I have fought a very hard battle, but I have also seen what strength I have inside of me. I have learned to appreciate all the things my body does for me, and I want to treat it nice… I am only 23 years old but I think I have learned many lessons other people don't learn during a lifetime, and most importantly I have learned to live in the present. I have learned to cherish each ray of sunshine that comes my way… I have learned that life is not that serious. That there should be room for playing in it. For laughter and for fun.

I won't go back there… Never ever. I have seen how it's like on the other side. And I am not willing to give up the colors in life, just to see a lower number on my scale. That's too high a price for too low living. I am not willing to pay that price. Not anymore. Life is so much more than the numbers on the scale.

Life can be fun!

By Shinyflower, 23. Nurse. Norway. Anorexia for 6 years. Recovered. If you want to get in touch with Shinyflower, send an e-mail to **lillebie@europe.com**.

Do you know how special and unique you are? That you really matter in this world. That someone has noticed you and care about you. That you make a huge difference in someone's life. Do you know that you are needed? Do you know that you are loved? Do you know that you are accepted?

I see all your pain and there is nothing I want more than to be able to take all your pain and sorrow away. I wish I could take your hearts in my hands and heal all your wounds. I wish I could make everything allright. I wish I could make you whole again. I wish I could take all your burdens on my shoulders and carry you in my arms until you feel strong enough to walk yourself. But I can't live your life for you. You have to fight the battle yourself. But there will be people beside you. You will make it.

Dare to believe that you are beautiful.

Dare to believe that you are unique

Dare to believe that you make a difference

Dare to believe that you are loved

Dare to believe that you are talented

Dare to believe that you have your own special way of reaching out to others.

Dare to believe that you have the right to be here.

Dare to believe that you have the right to take up space

Dare to believe that you can do it.

Dare to believe that you can spread your wings and fly

Dare to believe that you can feel good again

Dare to believe that everything will be allright

Dare to believe that no matter what have happened, things can be better

Dare to believe that your future is bright

Dare to believe that there is always hope.

Dare to believe that you will recover.

Dare to believe that you will live again

Because...

You ARE beautiful.

You ARE unique.

You DO make a difference.

You ARE loved

You ARE talented

You DO have your special way of reaching out to others

You DO have the right to be here.

You DO have the right to take up space.

You CAN do it.

You CAN spread your wings and fly...

You CAN feel good again.

Everything WILL be allright; it's only a matter of time.

The past doesn't matter, that's not the way you are going

As long as there is life, there IS hope.

You CAN recover, but it is up to you

You WILL live again.

You WILL shine.

You WILL radiate.

Dare to believe, because there can be miracles when you believe. And you are loved, no matter what the ed tells you. You are loved beyond understanding and words.

All of you are loved.
All of you are unique, something special.
All of you are a piece of a big puzzle.

By Shinyflower, 23. Nurse. Norway. Anorexia for 6 years. Recovered. If you want to get in touch with Shinyflower, send an e-mail to **lillebie@europe.com**.

My Psychosomatic Obsessive Disorder

By Vera Fleischer, 30. Germany. EDNOS (Eating Disorder Not Otherwise Specified) for 2 years. Depression. Diagnosed with Mental Illness and OCD (Obsessive Compulsive Disorder). Recovered

My Psychosomatic Obsessive Disorder: 4th Grade

In 4th grade I was happy as a clam. It was one of the best years of my life, as I remember it. I was getting A's for penmanship, I was popular in my class, and I had a lot of imagination. I was playful and creative, outspoken and funny. I had a crush on a boy in my class and I was pretty sure that he had a crush on me too, although I never did find out. I had my two best friends, Anna* and Melanie*, who lived on my street and were in my class as well. I had two parents and two siblings, and we lived in a house. There were 22 people in my class, and I knew all of their birthdays, and I loved our teacher, the lovely Frau Dömer-Brink. My life was perfectly in order.

That spring, a hint of neurosis made itself felt. I noticed that under no circumstances did I want to have diarrhea. Diarrhea was the absolute worst thing that could happen to me. This was the only time in my life where I would have rather vomited than had diarrhea. I was afraid to death of diarrhea. I started to obsess over getting diarrhea and how horrible that would be. Every day after school I obsessed about it to my mom, crying and freaking out because what if I got diarrhea? My mom asked me what was so bad about diarrhea. I said "Because it makes those noises!" My mom and dad thought it was funny that I said that but I was dead serious. I didn't think it was funny at all. We were talking about diarrhea after all, the worst thing that could happen to me!

I think what I was so afraid of was not having control over my body. I was afraid of not having control over the noises my body made and over the speed at which my poop came out. I desperately wanted to control those things. I think I was also afraid of being gross, making gross noises and having gross stuff come out of me.

One afternoon, when I would not stop freaking out about diarrhea, my mom called our pediatrician. I stopped screaming and listened. I was fascinated by her action. Hidden in this whole scene was a cry for attention. I don't know why I needed more attention but I think part of it was that my parents never took my "problems" seriously. Nothing truly bad had ever happened to me, so they didn't conceive that I could be upset about anything. Years before that I remember complaining that I didn't like my curly hair and that I didn't like my deep voice. All my mom could say in response to that was "You poor, poor child" in a mocking tone. When I was in the hospital with a neural disease at age 5, my dad, knowing that I had a tendency to complain about my unsatisfactory human condition, carried me around to show me the children in the intensive car unit that were hooked up to hoses and machines. He said "See those children? They have problems. You don't have problems."

Well, that day in 4th grade I was glad that my mom told the pediatrician that I had a problem. So I stopped screaming about diarrhea and listened to the conversation. She told him that it was more of a psychological than a physical problem. I was thrilled. I had a psychological problem! The pediatrician told my mom to give me a stool softener so that I would poop already, and if things didn't get better, he would give her the name of a psychiatrist.

I did calm down about diarrhea. I was still deathly afraid of it, but I stopped obsessing and screaming about it. One time I was at my grandparents' house, and when I walked by the bathroom with my grandma in it, I could hear that she had diarrhea. Or maybe she didn't have diarrhea and that's just how she pooped. But I remember thinking "How can she not freak out? Listen to that! I would die if that happened to me. My grandma is a brave lady."

Aside from that glitch, I went on with my happy 4th grade life. In the summer after 4th grade, I went to my first summer camp with all my friends, and I had the time of my life. I got to hang out with all these cool older people. Pretty older girls that wore hairspray! Cute older boys that were really funny! I was in heaven. But I did get diarrhea during summer camp. All my friends threw up, but I got diarrhea when the stomach flu went around. I panicked. And then I went to my favorite camp leader and told her that I had diarrhea and that I was really afraid of diarrhea and asked her if she would go to the bathroom with me so I wouldn't be so scared. She agreed. I went into one of the stalls while she waited by the sinks. I did my business. I asked her "Can you hear anything?" She lied "No." Even though I knew she was lying, I was eternally grateful for it. I didn't want anybody to acknowledge my gross and scary diarrhea noises.

My Psychosomatic Obsessive Disorder: Hospital Visits

After the diarrhea debacle, my family and I didn't know what we were in for. A big dark cloak enveloped our lives in the fall of 1986, the beginning of my 5th grade. Elementary school in Germany ends after 4th grade, and you have to choose from three types of secondary schools: Hauptschule ("Main School"), Realschule ("Intermediate School"), and Gymnasium ("High School"). The not-so-smart kids went to Hauptschule, the intermediate kids to Realschule, and the smart kids to Gymnasium. Nice segregation, right? I know. Everybody said I was smart, so I went to Gymnasium. My best friends Anna and Melanie went to Hauptschule. Did I mention how much I loved my elementary school class and my teacher? The only person from my class that ended up in my class at Gymnasium was Marko*. A boy! Do you know what this meant? It meant that I didn't have one friend in my new class. Changing from elementary to secondary school was the most traumatic thing that ever happened to me. It was worse than any lost friend, worse than any breakup, worse even than leaving behind my family and friends to move to another country. It was THAT BAD. Going to that new school in a new town was a problem for me, a big problem.

It wasn't apparent at first. It started out innocently enough. I felt I was ready to move on with my life and be a "big girl". A 5th grade High School girl. How exciting! But after about a month, I started obsessing again. I obsessed that nobody in my new class liked me. There was an odd number of girls in the class, and I was the only one who didn't have a "match." I obsessed that my old best friends, Anna and Melanie, who were together in the same class at the school for not-as-smart kids, didn't like me anymore. I obsessed that my parents didn't love me. But most importantly, I obsessed that I was fat. In particular, my belly was fat. My belly was so fat, I didn't deserve to live. I wanted to die. Elementary school was gone forever, my family didn't care about me, and my belly was fat. My life was over.

It was around this time that I first found out about anorexia. I had read about it and seen a film about it on TV. I decided that I wanted to be anorexic. The concept of being scarily skinny and even of being mentally ill really appealed to me. How tragic I would be! My parents would have to take my complaints and crying about life seriously. I knew that you could die from anorexia. "Even better!" I thought. "I'm about ready to die."

I told my parents that I wanted to die. I told my parents that I wanted to go on a diet. My parents told me that they loved me, and that I wasn't fat, and that surely I would make some new friends soon. But I wasn't having any of it. There was nothing they could have said to make me feel better. This became clear when one day in early October, I started raging. My mom went to a friend's house one afternoon and took me with her, but I stayed in the car and kicked the inside of the car the whole time she was inside her friend's house. The next day I screamed and kicked walls and threw things across my room. I broke stuff. My mom called the pediatrician again. Again I paused my raging and listened. She asked "Can 10-year-olds be depressed? I think she is depressed." I was thrilled. A mental disorder! That'll show them! The pediatrician told my mom to call a psychiatrist, Dr. Mayr* in Münster, near my dad's work. My dad came home from work early that day, with a serious look on his face, and they took me to see Dr. Mayr. I noticed that my mom had with her a bag full of my clothes. I asked her "Do I have to stay there?" She said maybe. I was calm on the way to the hospital. It was October 3, 1986. I stayed there for seven and a half weeks.

I talked to Dr. Mayr every day. I didn't like him very much because he was keeping me in the hospital, but I could tell that he was a nice man. My dad came to see me every day on his lunch break. Thinking about how he picked me up for a walk every day makes me cry to this day. I was at the psychosomatic children's ward. *Psychosomatic* was one of the biggest words in my vocabulary at that time. I knew it meant *mind-body*. I knew I had problems with my mind whose symptoms were directly related to my body because I was sad that I was fat. The other children at the psychosomatic ward were between 8 and 16. I was 10. I first shared a room with Hanna*, the youngest girl there. She always "had to lie." The day I got there, she told us that her birthday was the next day. The next day my mom brought her a present and got Hanna in trouble because it wasn't really her birthday. She had lied. Later I shared a room with 13-year-old Christine* who always "had to wash herself." See, I wasn't the only one who was obsessive-compulsive. There was also a younger girl named Daniela*. She couldn't eat. Then there were several girls between 14 and 16 who were anorexic. They were all very skinny and I admired them all. I looked up to them. The father of one of the anorexic girls, Monika*, worked for the same company as my dad. I admired Monika a lot. She had beautiful handwriting.

I didn't like being at the hospital. I wanted to go home. I wanted to have my freedom back. I threatened Dr. Mayr that I would run away, and he threatened me with a locked ward. I also threatened him that I would stop eating because I was fat, and he threatened me with a feeding tube. I knew it hurt a lot to have a feeding tube put through your nose and throat. The other girls had told me. He didn't really threaten me. He just mentioned the locked ward and the feeding tube as "alternatives." I didn't like some of the questions he asked me. I felt he was insinuating that I was full of crap. I didn't like being accused of just wanting attention even though that was partially true.

There were several social workers who worked at the hospital. I liked and respected them. They were all in their 20's, the Birkenstock type. But I didn't like some of the questions they asked me either or the activities they made me do. I didn't like them making me play with instruments, do gymnastics, draw and paint, etc. I didn't want to play and be creative. That part of Vera had died when elementary school had ended, didn't they know that? But I did like jumping on the trampoline. Looking back, I don't understand why they didn't just let me jump on the trampoline all the time since I clearly liked it.

One time one of the social workers and I had a play date and were playing post office. I decided to write a post card to my mom. I wrote "Dear Mama, how are you? I'm doing badly..." The social worker asked why I didn't tell my mom that I was doing well. "Because I'm not!" I said. "I'm very unhappy." Then she said that if I told my mom that I was doing badly, she might worry about me, is that what I wanted? Yes, that's what I wanted. I was in the mental hospital, and I was fat and unhappy. My mom had every reason to worry about me, and I most certainly wanted her to. I didn't like that the social worker was insinuating that it was wrong of me to want my mom to worry about me.

I went to school during my stay at the hospital. It was a special part-time school for long-term hospital patients. Only the main subjects were taught - Latin and Math, and I remember being in an art class. I told every single teacher how miserable I was and that my parents didn't love me. I'm sure they thought I was a delight.

I had good days and bad days at the hospital. It was a good day when I stood on the edge of the bath tub and my belly looked flat in the mirror. It was a bad day when I stood on the edge of the bath tub and my belly looked big. On some days I had feelings of total bliss. They were accompanied by thoughts like "One day I will get out of here", "One day I will be happy again", "One day I will have my life back." And on other days I felt hopeless and stuck. I didn't want to be sick anymore and longed so much for everything to go back to the way it was. I wanted to go back to the way things were in 4th grade. But I knew that was impossible. I was in 5th grade now. And I was sick.

One time while I was at the hospital, I obsessed that my mom was going to die. Suddenly the possibility that she might die seemed very real to me, and I panicked. I told one of the nurses that I had to call my mom and make sure that she is okay. A social worker went outside to the phone booth with me and said that I could call my mom only on the condition that I didn't freak out. Of course the first thing I did when I had my mom on the phone was freak out. I started crying and screaming because what if she died? Then I wouldn't have a mom! The money ran out in the phone booth, and of course I wasn't allowed to call again. I couldn't sleep that night because I thought that my mom was going to die. I got up in the middle of the night and told the night nurse that I had to call my mom. But he said no.

Another time, on one of our excursions into town with a social worker and some of the other kids, we ran into my beloved elementary school teacher. She knew that I was in the hospital, and I knew that she knew, but neither of us said anything about that. We talked for a minute or so about meaningless stuff. More than anything in the world I wanted her to take me home with her and say that I could come back to elementary school, and that she would tell all the other kids from our 4th grade class to come back too. But I knew that she had a new 1st grade class now.

I was released from the hospital on November 21. My dad's birthday is on November 23, and he said that my coming home was his favorite birthday present. We all thought that things were going to be better from now on. But they weren't. I was still terribly sick and unhappy. The day after Christmas, I was upset about something--I don't remember what—and I ran out of the house without a jacket. I just took off running. There was a thick layer of snow everywhere. The worst part about this is that my mom put on her coat, grabbed my coat, and ran after me. She ran after me for a good half hour or so, but I was faster. At some point, we passed somebody we knew, I think, first me, than my mom. I don't even want to know what they must have thought. Finally my mom shouted "Vera, please stop! Let's go home, please! I can't do this anymore!" And I stopped. I put on the coat my mom had brought for me and we walked home together. The image of my mom running after me will haunt me for the rest of my life. It breaks my heart to think about what I put her through that day. I feel terrible for many, many things I did to my family during this time.

One day I decided to walk home from school the minute the bus dropped me off there. I had told my mom many times that I hated school because I didn't have any friends there and that I wanted to go back to elementary school. That morning I announced to my mom that I was going to walk home. I walked through snow and ice. It took me two hours and twenty minutes. Around 10am I rang the door bell at my parents' house, and my mom answered the door with a serious look on her face. "Hello Vera" she said with a sad voice. The next day the director of my school called me into his office. He wanted to know what was going on. Why had I walked home from school? I told him that I hated school because everybody hated me there. I also told him that my parents hated me and were really mean to me. I told him that I thought I was adopted because they clearly didn't want me. The director of my school was very concerned and called my parents in for a meeting. Luckily they were able to convince him that they did in fact love me very much, and that, outside of my skewed perception, they were very nice people.

Was I done humiliating and torturing my parents? No. Sometime in late January, I woke up in the morning and started raging again. My rage was directed toward my dad in particular. I don't even remember what I said, but it was something about him being such a horrible and mean person, and that he didn't love me, and that it was all his fault, and on and on. My dad was trying to have breakfast and get ready for work, and I just kept on raging. Finally, my dad hunched over in his chair and started sobbing. Just like that. There he was, my dad, sobbing, because of something I had said. I had made my dad cry. Who was the mean one now? I stopped raging and started crying. I couldn't believe I had done that and felt terrible. To this day, I cannot think about this incident without starting to cry. It is probably the most painful of all my painful memories, and I don't know how the universe can ever forgive me for what I did. I had made my own dad cry, my strong and mean dad. The only time I had ever seen him cry before that was at my great grandma's funeral.

The day I made my dad cry, my parents called Dr. Mayr, and I ended up back at the hospital. I stayed there for another three and a half weeks until sometime in February. This was my first case of the February Blues, my now almost annual gloomy friend. Some of the kids I already knew from the hospital were still there (like Christine, I think), but many of them were new. There was a 17-year-old guy named Markus*, and he was afraid to death of throwing up. He hadn't thrown up in six years and wanted to achieve the world record in not throwing up. I could relate because I was afraid to death of diarrhea. One time I asked Markus what he was writing. He told me that Dr. Mayr had asked him to write his life story. I asked Dr. Mayr later if he wanted me to write my life story too. He said that he doesn't usually ask patients as young as me to do that. I was disappointed. I wanted to write my life story, but since I wasn't instructed to do so, I didn't. There was also a 16-year-old anorexic girl whose name I forgot. She and Markus became a couple. Then there was Tobias*, 14. He wore cowboy boots. He told me that one of the guys from the locked ward, who rode the bus to the hospital school with us, was in the locked ward because he had killed somebody. Tobias scared me. Later on I would have dreams about him hurting my mom. I never found out what he was in the hospital for. I think he was too cool and tough to talk about it.

I'm pretty sure that this time I had my own room, though I don't remember why. But I do remember that the psychosomatic children's hospital is a sad, sad place to be, except for maybe the love birds Markus and the girl whose name I forgot.

I exchanged addresses with some of the girls, this time as well as the first time. Sandra*, an anorexic girl with a feeding tube who didn't eat but chain-smoked and drank lots of coffee, sent me letters on baby blue paper on which she drew beautifully shaped hearts, one bigger than the next. I once wrote a letter to the anorexic girl whose name I forgot asking her how much she had eaten when she had lost all that weight. She wrote me back with her exact diet and told me not to try this UNDER ANY CIRCUMSTANCES. Little did she know that I didn't have the willpower to be truly anorexic. I never did become anorexic. I just had this weird psychosomatic obsessive disorder with no name.

My Psychosomatic Obsessive Disorder: Bodies and Soul

One afternoon in 1986 I ate a Zwieback (a kind of crispbread) with butter on it. And then, just for fun and because it tasted so good, I had another one. My mom said "Watch out. If you keep eating like that, you'll rise like a pancake." I thought "Huh."

Another day, my friend Melanie was over and I told her that I thought my stomach was big. She said she didn't think that it was big. I said that it was definitely bigger than hers. She said "Maybe, but that doesn't mean it's big." I stood up, turned so she could see me sideways, and lifted my shirt. I breathed deeply into my stomach and pushed it all the way out and said "Look! That's how big it is. Doesn't it look like I'm pregnant?" Melanie said "Wow. When you do it like that, it does look a little bit like you're pregnant." And that's when I started sucking in my stomach, and to this day I still have to remind myself not to because it's so deeply programmed, now after almost 20 years.

My friends Melanie's and Anna's bodies were different from mine. I had brown hair; they were both blond. I wore glasses; they didn't. They were both petite--short and thin. I was tall and not really thin. I was pretty much exactly normal, whatever that means. I was by no means chubby or fat. You could call me slender, but you couldn't really me skinny. I was normal. But Anna and Melanie were skinny. I wanted to be skinny too. I didn't want to be normal anymore.

I tried to diet but I didn't really have enough willpower to go through with it. The temptation of food was stronger than my desire to be thin and it kept roping me back to join the eating masses. I kept trying to stop eating though, just like the real anorexics. I liked the idea of my parents worrying about me not eating enough. I once asked my mom "Are you ever worried that I'm not eating enough?" She said no, she wasn't really worried about that. I was disappointed. I got down on myself for not being strong enough to pull it through. If

I really managed to stop eating, somebody would surely worry about me sooner or later.

The truth is that everybody did worry about me. My family was worried sick about me. Not because I wasn't eating (because I was) but because I was just so sad. Around Christmas or so my grandma on my dad's side squeezed me tight against her big bosom and said "We can't have our girl be so sad! It's making us all sad that you're so sad!" She had tears in her eyes.

I cried every day. I had lost all interest in life. I had lost all interest in everything I enjoyed before. I didn't want to play. I didn't want to do art or crafts. I did play the piano though, especially this piece called Püppchens Begräbnis ("The funeral of the little doll") because it was really dark and somber and sad. And I read a lot of books. I read sad books, to be exact. Books about a 9-year-old girl dying from a brain tumor, books about an 11-year-old boy committing suicide, books about World War II, books about kids who were adopted, books about autistic kids, books about girls with anorexia. I loved reading books that made me cry. Crying about somebody else's life felt so good. I could do it for hours. Maybe it was because I wasn't allowed to cry about myself. My parents were always trying to get me to stop. They didn't like it when I cried. Only my grandma on my mom's side understood my need to cry. She had been treated for depression before, and she told me that sometimes she felt really good after crying, that crying helped her. Truth be told though, crying didn't really help me. It didn't make my belly any smaller.

My mom regularly took me to the library to pick out books to read. I think she was worried that I was always reading sad books. The woman working at the library always had suggestions for me. In her carroty voice she would tell me about *The Lord of the Rings* and *The Little Hobbit*, and just how fantastic these fantasy books were. I told her every time "I don't like that. Do you have any books about children who are mentally ill?"

My mom wanted me to get excited about life again. One day after school, the music teacher from my old elementary school, Frau Bauer*, stopped by. She told me that she was leading the girls' scouts in our town and asked me if I would like to join. I said "No, definitely not." My mom came to the door as well. I knew suddenly that my mom had asked Frau Bauer to stop by. I said "No, I don't want to join the girls' scouts." My mom and Frau Bauer both looked said and concerned, and Frau Bauer left.

Anna and Melanie were still my friends. But they admitted that what was going on with me was a little bit weird. They also admitted that they didn't really know how to deal with it or what to do about my sadness. I translated that to them not wanting me anymore. One time early on, when my disease was just starting to surface, I remember being with Anna at a brook in the neighborhood. We looked at the water and the sticks and stones. Anna said something about one of the stones. She felt so innocent in that moment, and what we were doing was so innocent. But I knew that we were growing up, and the older kids were starting to influence us. There was fashion and music and popularity. There were social rules and ways to be cool and ways to be uncool. I could feel all of that encroaching on our innocent girlhood and friendship. I just wanted us to stay the way we were forever, just two little girls by a brook, innocent, childlike and loving each other unconditionally. But I could feel it slipping away, and along with it I could feel Anna starting to slip away. It made my heart ache hard.

I also made some new friends at school. Everybody liked me, really, they were just a little bit concerned because I was always so sad and always thinking about what I was eating. One time I was at a birthday party at somebody's house, and Sonja* later told everybody that she had used the bathroom after me, and that she could tell that I had made myself throw up. The truth is that I never made myself throw up. I was too chicken to do it. And I hated Sonja for spreading lies about me. I was trying very hard to be anorexic, yes, but I was not bulimic.

At school we had this box called the "sorrow box." Once a week we would open it to find notes from anybody in class who was concerned about anything. I frequently entered notes that said things like "Nobody likes me" or "Judith R.* gave some licorice to other girls, but not to me." One time at a birthday party, we were having a big group girl talk. I brought up some of my insecurities that I was feeling with respect to the other girls. But I was quickly told that it made everybody very uncomfortable when I did that, so I never did anything like that again for almost 20 years.

Sven*, my elementary school buddy and neighbor, was in the class next door to mine at the new school. He told me that one of the teachers had told his whole class about me and that I was sick and that everybody should be nice to me. I was embarrassed by how public my issues were, but at the same time I enjoyed the attention.

There was a period of time in the spring of 1987 when I actually lost some weight. You have to understand that in Germany, lunch is the biggest meal, and dinner is small and not much different from breakfast. And I just ate a light lunch. I ate like this for several months, I think, and lost some pounds.

In times when I didn't have enough willpower to be on a strict diet, I still kept a food journal and counted my calories. My mom had this little booklet from a magazine that listed the calories for common foods. The calories were usually listed for a 100g serving. Sometimes I weighed my food on a food scale, and sometimes I just lifted my pasta off of my plate with my hand, estimating how much it weighed. My sister once asked me why I was lifting my pasta, and I reluctantly and embarrassedly told her that I was weighing it. Sometimes I would ask my mom "How many calories do you think this sandwich has?" She could never give me the right answer, although she certainly did try. If she estimated a low number, I accused her of trying to get me fat. If she estimated a high number, I accused of her not allowing me to eat. My mom sure had a difficult job.

When trying not to eat, my desire for food only grew stronger and stronger. I soon noticed that I could eat and eat and eat, and then I could eat some more. At night in bed I started fantasizing about eating chocolate cake and pudding and fruit gummies and pizza and lots of ice cream and whipped cream and.. One time I bragged to my dad that I could eat more than he could. He said "Oh yeah?" I said "Yeah. I could eat TEN sandwiches." We agreed that I would prove it to him. The next morning for breakfast I ate ten sandwiches. I could have kept going, but the deal was to eat ten. I enjoyed it because it gave me an excuse to eat. And my parents enjoyed it because it gave me an excuse to eat.

I also weighed myself several times a day. And I monitored the status of my belly in the mirror. I either used the mirror in the lobby, a very central location in our house, or I stood on our bath tub (just like I did in the hospital) and used the bathroom mirror. Either way, I would drop my pants to my ankles, lift my shirt and then look at my belly from all angles. One time, my neighbor Sven asked me "Did you stand in front of the mirror naked the other day?" I lied "No" and was more careful about the windows being covered going forward.

At the end of 5th grade, I went to summer camp again. I was happy again, just like the year before. For the first time in almost a year, I felt like myself again. I laughed a lot and goofed around. Everybody that saw me in camp that summer could tell that I was happy again. But that didn't mean that I was actually better. When school continued in 6th grade, it all started up again.

My Psychosomatic Obsessive Disorder: 6th Grade

In 6th grade I wasn't suicidal anymore but I was still obsessed with food and being thin. And my general dissatisfaction with life persisted. And I developed a new obsession. It was about wealth. In 6th grade I became aware that the parents of some of my new friends at school were very wealthy. I might have known wealthy people before but I hadn't seen this kind of wealth with these kinds of houses. Andrea's* father owned a factory. She had her own horse, and her family lived in a huge house with a grand piano and stairs as big as the ones at our school. Claudia's* father was a chiropractor with his own practice. They lived in a very big and very stylish white house with a round window, a huge backyard with a pond and a little river, and a swimming pool in the basement. Karin's* father owned an antique furniture store. They lived in a huge house with an alarm system and expensive antique furniture everywhere. My family lived in a small one-story house with no alarm, pool, or antique furniture. Luckily, popularity in our class wasn't dependent on your parents' wealth. But I still noticed that these girls' families were wealthy, and mine wasn't. I also noticed that some of the girls in my class were wearing certain brand names I had never heard of before. Those brands were, in order of importance, Oilily, Esprit and Benetton. I became obsessed with having to have Oilily clothes.

My mom wouldn't have been caught dead buying us Oilily clothes. One of her main goals in life was to spend as little money on stuff as possible. Sometimes she knitted and sewed clothes for us because it was cheaper that way. And now I was making demands for Oilily clothes, which were about three times more expensive than my mom was used to spending.

After much arguing, pleading and screaming, my parents agreed to buy me a beautiful pair of pink Oilily pants, the most expensive piece of clothing I or my mom had ever owned. Claudia had blue Oilily pants and a pink and red Oilily sweatshirt that looked great together. I had pink Oilily pants and a generic pink sweatshirt, but still! I loved my Oilily pants. But I soon wanted more and started screaming again.

My dad said that he would gladly buy me all the Oilily I wanted if he knew that it would make me happy. But he said that he didn't think that all the clothes in the world would make me happy. I would find something else to be unhappy about. I had to admit that he was right. But I still wanted Oilily.

For Christmas, my mom and I found a blue Oilily coat that was on sale. It was still heinously expensive, but it was over 50% off of its original price. Karin had the same coat in red. I had to have it. My mom bought it for me for Christmas. I was so excited; I took the coat to bed with me that night.

But I still wanted more. I was obsessed. I looked at everybody I encountered to see if they were wearing Oilily or some other brand name. I started mentally putting people in the "wealthy" and "not wealthy" categories. I told my parents that I thought they should be more wealthy. I told them I was ashamed that our family wasn't wealthier. I told my mom to get a job so that we would have more money. I'm sure I hurt them a lot.

That year my parents bought us a dog. Her name was Sheila and she was a very cute puppy. I loved her, but I was also wishing that she had been pure bred and more expensive. I think one of the reasons my parents got her is that they were hoping a dog would make me happy again. And it did, for about a day. Just like the Oilily pants.

I complained to my parents that we didn't have a wealthy enough lifestyle. We lived in a house that was too small; we didn't fly on vacation but drove; we had generic store-brand chocolate bars, not the fancy brand kind. My dad took me to a four star hotel for a night, just me and him. I really appreciated the gesture and had a good time, but I still wasn't happy. Our family still wasn't wealthy.

While in 5th grade I was sad and angry, in 6th grade I was jealous and greedy. Jealous of other people's wealth, greedy for my own wealth, and nasty to my family. One time we watched a documentary about a heroin addict who was prostituting herself until a rich man fell in love with her and rescued her away from the streets and the drug. She was now married to a rich man. I said to my parents "Maybe I'll do some heroin so I can get rich too." My dad got angry and told me that money wasn't everything. He said that I had a sister and a brother and I should be thankful for that. I said that I would rather have a lot of money than a sister and a brother. He said that I should be ashamed of myself, and I was. I still am. I'm ashamed of the money-hungry monster I turned into at age 11.

I don't know how my parents continued to love me after all that, but somehow they did. I think many times during those two years, they told themselves that the little monster that was living in their house wasn't really me, but my mental illness.

My Psychosomatic Obsessive Disorder: Coming Out Of It

During the two years in which I had my psychosomatic obsessive disorder, I had several smaller obsessions that I won't mention and don't even remember. But one of them played an important role in me finally getting better. It was the obsession over waking up too early in the morning. I am and always have been a morning person. I usually wake up naturally between 7 and 8am. This became a problem for me when I was trying to diet. On weekends I usually woke up earlier than the rest of my family, and the first thing I wanted to do in the morning was eat something. (I am still like that today, by the way. If I don't eat something within an hour or so of waking up, I start feeling uncomfortably hungry.) So I would get myself something to eat, but then an hour or so later, the rest of my family would get up and have a big family breakfast, and I would want to join them for that. But then I would eat breakfast twice. And since I was trying to diet, that was unacceptable. I dreaded waking up on the weekends out of fear of waking up too early. I started obsessing over my wake up time, and it became like a sport for me. If I ever slept until 9 or 10, I was super happy. Sometimes I obsessed about it the night before, and it ruined my night. I was tired and wanted to go to bed, but I was so afraid that I would wake up too early the next morning that I forced myself to stay awake, but then I was miserably tired. And sometimes I even cried about it. On some Friday or Saturday nights I cried because I knew that I would wake up so early the next morning that I would end up eating breakfast twice, and then I would be fat.

In the spring of 1988, towards the end of my 6th grade, my family went on vacation in Austria to ski. The second or so day that we were there, I started freaking out again about waking up too early the next day, and I started crying. My parents were frustrated because they were trying to enjoy their vacation. My dad told me that I had to stop crying about something that hadn't even happened yet. He said that if I woke up too early the next morning, I could still cry then. But if I continued to cry about it the night before when it hasn't even happened yet, our vacation was over and he would take us all back home. I stopped crying because I really wanted to stay in Austria and ski.

I don't know what time I woke up the next morning. But when I woke up that morning, I was healed. I could feel that I was happy again. I knew that the mental illness was gone, all of it. What my dad had said to me the night before had shifted something in me. Something finally got through to my head and made me realize that I had a choice to obsess over things and be miserable, or to not obsess over things and be okay. So I stopped all of my obsessing.

I finally started seeing that I wasn't fat and did not need to lose any weight. I did insist though that if I ever did get fat, I would be very upset. But that hadn't happened yet, so I was okay NOW. And look at that, 18 years later I'm still not fat!

The next time I saw Dr. Mayr I told him that I was healed. He believed me. I saw him a few more times just to be sure, the last one being shortly after 7th grade started. I even brought him a book I had made: My creativity was back too. 7th grade went on to be totally awesome. I made lots of new friends at school and was my old funny, boisterous and energetic self again. I was back!

By Vera Fleischer, 30. Germany. EDNOS (Eating Disorder Not Otherwise Specified) for 2 years. Depression. Diagnosed with Mental Illness and OCD (Obsessive Compulsive Disorder). Recovered. For more information, please go to www.verabug.com.

* Name has been changed to protect person's privacy.

My Road To Recovery

By Stephanie, 20. Arizona, USA. Anorexia for 6 years. Self-Harm. Survivor of Sexual Abuse and Rape. Recovered.

It's easy to think when things get hard that I'm too sad to eat, or too upset to care about food. It's still a struggle at times to correct that thought, to actively tell myself that giving in to those old habits will only create more problems, that it will be even harder to correct next time if I let this once slide. I tried to make the decision to work for my health several times, and each time I started off strong, determined, and stubborn, but my resolve would fade, I'd doubt myself and my strength, and I'd lose faith in myself and let go of that decision. After a few attempts, the people around me lost faith in me, too, and that became one more trial in the road to recovery.

Another aspect that made it difficult was that I hated that those around me – doctors, therapists, family, friends – were trying to control in me what I couldn't, and I wanted to fight them and do it myself. Well, how do you fight against people trying to help you when secretly and honestly you want the same thing? I had to accept that this was my thing. They could do what they wanted, but ultimately this was my battle, my responsibility to fight. They could try to help me, but I was the only one who could do the work.

At the time there were two main reasons for my decision (again) to try to get my health back; try to get my life back: (a) I wanted with a burning passion to prove everyone telling me I was too weak to do it myself wrong, and (b) I missed who I was when I was happy and healthy, not to mention I missed my freedom. I stopped comparing myself physically to the people around me, forced myself to focus on their faces, eyes, on something other than their bodies. I stopped going to the online sites, including many support sites, because there were just too many triggering messages on them. If Ana wanted to be jealous of the ones who were suffering even more than I was, then I was going to prevent myself and it from seeing any others. I'd tried scaring myself out of an eating disorder, and the only thing it had done was make me strive to get closer, so that was out. A difficult thing as I started to put on weight was the reactions of those around me.

Comments about looking healthier, about looking different, in my mind automatically translated to "looking heavier". *Untrue*, I said. *What they are seeing is the color returning to me, what they are seeing is my eyes looking alive, my hair no longer looking dull, feeling my skin warm for the first time* – I was the only one who knew I was gaining weight, everyone around me saw only something new, some new life somehow in me.

If the first week was hard, the second week was harder. Therapists telling me and my mother that I was just putting on weight to get them off my back that they could see through me. Nutritionists changing their minds on the weight they wanted me at, increasing it for a "safety layer" of pounds. I threw my tantrums at them, angry that they couldn't appreciate what I was doing and be grateful that in their eyes I was cooperating. But it was useless; I was too stubborn to give in at this point. After all, if I gave in, I would prove them all right, I would prove to them that this had all been an act, that I was too weak, that I had once again failed to live. The more they told me they could see through me, the more I knew I had to get better. If they were going to tell me I couldn't do it without their help, I was going to prove to everyone and myself that I was stronger than any of them had imagined. In the long run, it was more important that I was proving my strength to myself, and I wish I could say it was at the time as important as I know it is now, but when I was in that moment, I was just the underdog trying to show the world and make a point. After the second week, I started counting the weeks I had been eating normally. Three weeks, four weeks, five. At eight weeks, my closest friends threw me a party. It was little victories in my battle for life.

As time passed, the real foundation for my recovery began to be laid. I started to realize that recovering wasn't about proving everyone around me wrong – it was about me, and my life, and my future. It was about re-defining the things in my life, prioritizing reasonably – did I want to be thin, or did I want to live? No more of this 'I'd rather die than gain weight'. That wasn't true. I was scared of dying, and yet all this time I'd been trying to slowly starve myself to death? Facing life was a terrifying concept for sure, getting better was something that seemed larger than life, that from within a psychiatric unit seemed more than impossible. But at least I had an idea of what life was. I had an inkling of what life could be, yet I had been so willing to turn in fear from that and jump headfirst into death – something that no one knows for sure about.

The reasons and causes of Ana surfaced little by little, events and ideas that I'd never entertained as problems that now required some other way of coping. Recovery was best described as a learning process. Physically it was a challenge; putting on weight, feeling different, it was hard to adjust to, and I had a lot to learn and accept about being healthy. The hardest thing was the thought-processes. I was pretty sure they were there to stay forever. As the weeks went by (I counted through week 96, by the way), I developed a way of outthinking the thoughts, of talking myself into health as opposed to Ana. But when I saw someone I recognized as having an eating disorder, it was hard not to let go and start competing again. It took a lot to remind myself that that was not a path I wanted to go down again. After a little over a year, the doctors appointments and therapy appointments ended; therapy because I had never participated, and weigh-ins because I had shown I was capable of staying healthy. My family was still a little skeptical, even to this day I get questions about my eating, but I can accept now that they are not doubting me, just showing me that they remember it's hard. Today I can appreciate their concern, instead of spitefully considering it a personal insult. But, back to the thoughts. They are the hardest part, because they are so consistent. They were always there in the back of my mind, waiting for a moment of weakness to try to re-instate themselves. Three years after I had decided to fight for my health and my happiness, while I was traveling to a new school in Arizona, I realized one day that the entire day had passed without any trace of guilt or those thoughts. I thought back a little more, and couldn't remember any time from the previous day either, and not only that, but I felt like I was finally starting to see things for what they really were. I looked at myself in the mirror in my bathing suit on my way out to the pool, and I liked what I saw. It was a very strange feeling, one that I couldn't honestly say I'd had before. All throughout my recovery, as I struggled to gain the weight, fought against my own mind, tried to regain the trust and faith of everyone around me, every time I won some of my life back I knew everything I was going through was worth it. But not one of those little victories compared to that moment. I had figured I would always be "in recovery", that it would never really go away. Today I still get those desires to compete, mostly when I am having a bad day or rough time and see someone or hear something that I recognize as somehow related to Ana, and there is just this instantaneous flash of emotion, that intense controlling competitive feeling. In that sense I think that there is always a part of Ana in me, not because I wasn't strong enough to forget it completely, but just because it's a part of me, it's a part of my past. To me the greater thing is that I *feel* recovered now. At that moment when I was completely content with what I saw in the mirror, I decided that that must be what it meant to be "recovered", that when I could look around and recognize that I was happy being healthy, that truly I wanted life more than I ever wanted to give in to Ana, that was recovered to me.

By Stephanie, 20. Arizona, USA. Anorexia for 6 years. Self-Harm. Survivor of Sexual Abuse and Rape. Recovered.

Finding My True Self and Inner Beauty

By Andrea Roe, 24, Austrian. Married to a wonderful Canadian. Currently living in Langley, British Columbia, Canada. Anorexia for 2 years. Bulimia for 4 years. Depression. Recovered.

My name is Andrea. I am 24 years old and a recovered anorexic and bulimic. I am Austrian, married to a wonderful Canadian and am currently living in Langley, British Columbia, Canada. I struggled with eating disorders for six long years and have finally overcome these deadly diseases – and this is my story...

While I was growing up, food and weight were not a problem for me. I come from a very active and health-oriented family and never had to worry about my weight. Almost every weekend my parents would take my siblings and me walking, hiking, biking, skiing or on a sightseeing trip to a gorgeous place somewhere in Austria. I like thinking about my childhood; it was a wonderful time and thinking about it creates a warm feeling inside of me. Even now, while I am writing this, I have a smile on my face and a tear of joy in my eyes.

When I was about thirteen years old, someone said to me that my smile was ugly, that my face looked weird when I smiled and then she started to laugh. She said this in front of other people. I was very confused; I did not know what to say and I blushed. I had never paid much attention to my smile until that day. When I came home from school, I looked at myself in the mirror. I smiled. I used two mirrors and looked at my smile at different angles. I stared at myself for hours and came to the conclusion that this girl was right: My smile was ugly! I looked ugly when I smiled. And on this day I decided not to smile anymore. It took me almost ten years till I learnt to love my smile again. On the pictures that were taken during these years, I hardly ever smiled. This happened about three years before my eating disorder developed but it was the first step towards disliking and hating my face and eventually my body.

Around this time, my skin started to get unclear too and I developed acne. I already did not like my face because of my 'ugly' smile and having unclear skin made me hate my face even more. I tried everything that was on the market to get rid of my skin problem but nothing helped me. I became depressed and cried a lot.

I started wearing make up to cover up the red spots on my face. I would not leave the house without putting it on – so ashamed I was of my face. There were times when I did not go to school because of my skin – I didn't want anyone to look at it. I did not like people looking at me, at my skin – I did not want them to look at what was 'wrong' with me.

My parents did everything in their power to help, support and comfort me – they were always there for me. I had times where I cried almost every day and locked myself in my room. I just wanted to be alone. I would lie on my bed, look at my face in a mirror and cry. I don't think many people knew about these struggles and how big of a problem my skin really was for me. I was a very sad teenage girl on the inside, but did not show this to other people. I pretended to be strong.

On my quest to find my 'cure', I learned that what one eats also has an effect on one's skin. That was a very interesting and appealing concept for me and I read every book about this topic that I got my hands on. I went on a strict diet and only ate 'good' food – 'good food' being healthy food that was supposed to be beneficial for the skin. This way of eating had nothing whatsoever to do with weight control – it was only about my skin. I was on this diet for almost a year but nothing changed. My skin was still disgusting and I still looked ugly. I felt so discouraged, helpless and hopeless and I cried even more than I did before. Many times I thought I would have to look like this for the rest of my life and I just had to learn to accept it and learn to live with it.

My best friend back then was a very gorgeous girl. In my eyes, she had it all – a beautiful face, clear skin, a slim and tone body and an open personality. She was just amazing and perfect in my eyes – the most beautiful girl! I couldn't stop comparing myself with her. She was everything I was not – at least that is what I thought. She was the gorgeous beauty, and I was the ugly beast. When I compared myself with her I felt worthless and ugly. I felt unseen. Invisible.

At some point, I must have been around fifteen or sixteen years old, I had this thought in my head that I had to lose some weight around my hips. I was never overweight by any means; I was always pretty slim – but never as slim as my best friend. So I began experimenting with diets – but I was still in control of my eating habits. At this point, I didn't even know what an eating disorder was. I don't know exactly when my eating disorder started and my dieting ended… I just slipped into it.

Over time I developed anorexia. I obsessively watched what I ate. I read a lot of women magazines and adored the women in those magazines – their beautiful smiles, their clear skin and their flawless bodies. Back then I did not know that what I looked at, what I admired and wanted to look like, was not real but digitally airbrushed and drastically altered by computers. At this point, I did not know that I had a problem. I was in denial and thought that what I was doing was normal. Now, when I look back, I can see how much I was already in my eating disorder world. I just did not notice it back then.

A lot of boys I knew had a crush on my best friend. She was one of these people that would enter a room and everybody would look at her. Wherever she went she got noticed. And then there was me…. Ugly smile, unclear skin, and shy. I am not sure if there were boys who liked me, but back then I did not feel as if any guy was interested. And why should they have been? There was nothing special or beautiful about me. At least that's what I thought.

I was the only one of my friends who did not have a boyfriend. And I felt weird about it. This was proof for me that there was indeed something wrong with me – and I knew exactly what it was: It must have been because I was ugly; it must have been because of my smile and my skin.

Sometimes, when lying in bed at night, I imagined what it would be like if I was like my best friend. How 'easy' life would be because I would not have to hide anymore. I wouldn't have to be afraid of people looking at me anymore – I could be free of all my worries! I thought I would be happy…

After graduating at the age of 18, I went to university. My former best friend and I went separate ways but the idea of me not being beautiful was still stuck in my head. And it was at this point that my eating disorder started to take complete control over my life, as well.

I started binging in order to try and fill the emptiness inside of me – though I never threw up. I wanted to so much, but for some reason I was not able to make myself vomit. I guess I was scared of it in a way. Instead, I would use other methods to get rid of the food and the calories quickly. I would eat till my stomach started to ache. I felt disgusted by myself and what I was doing. I was very ashamed and embarrassed of my behaviour. For the longest time I did not tell anyone about my problem and struggled on my own, secretly and in silence.

Unfortunately, my eating disorder didn't stop there. Not only did it change my relationship with food and weight – now, it started taking control over my social life as well. I didn't go out for a coffee, lunch or dinner with my friends anymore. I felt uncomfortable eating in front of other people. I didn't want anyone to force me to eat. I was terrified by the thought of gaining weight. I also feared that they would notice what was going on with me. I was afraid of them asking questions. I did not want anyone to find out what I was doing and lied a lot to my friends in order to keep my eating disorder secret. I did not like lying to them but I felt I had no other choice. I thought that if they knew they wouldn't like me anymore and wouldn't want to be friends with me anymore.

During the first couple of years of my struggles, I was not very educated about eating disorders – mainly because I was in denial for so long. I knew some basic information but not a lot. I also had no idea about where to get useful information about eating disorders, where to turn for help – I was too shy to ask. I thought that one has to be either extremely skinny or extremely heavy in order to be taken seriously. But I was never extremely skinny or extremely heavy. My weight was always somewhere in the normal healthy weight range. And don't people with eating disorders have to be one of those extremes?

I eventually hit a point where I could not deny my problem any longer and was finally able to admit to myself that what I was doing was not healthy and that I needed to stop this behaviour. But I did not know what to do, where to start… I felt lost, confused and thought I was the only one who had this problem.

I began reading eating disorder books, but nothing helped me. None of what I was reading was able to get through to me and make me stop what I was doing. And what was I doing? I was ruining not only my mind and health, I was ruining my life. I was hurting not only myself but also the people around me. Many nights I would cry myself to sleep, wondering if I was ever going to recover – or if there even was such a thing as 'recovery'.

I always had a very close relationship with my parents but my eating disorder forced me to move away from them. I became very reserved and quiet. They knew what was going on, and hoped that I would talk to them so they could support and help me. Sometimes I wanted to tell them what was going on, I wanted to be taken in their arms, wanted to feel that I was loved no matter what. I thought about talking to them for months but I was never sure of what to say. I was afraid of disappointing my parents. I wanted them to be proud of me. But how can they be proud of me when I have an eating disorder?

I eventually opened up to my mum. I gave her a book about how to deal with someone who struggles with an eating disorder, and I wrote a letter to her as well. I could see how relieved she was that I finally opened up to her, and she took me in her arms and comforted me. I was crying a lot on that day but I was glad I told her.

My eating disorder didn't get better after the conversation I had with my mum, but at least I knew now that I had someone to talk to when I needed help, comfort and support.

After I told my mum I went to a therapist. The therapist I went to was not specialized on eating disorders – she was a general therapist. I was so nervous about calling her and it took me a couple of days till I was ready to call her office and set up an appointment.

My appointment was on a sunny afternoon some time in spring. I was 19 years old. I remember sitting in her office and telling her my life story. She sat opposite of me on the other side of the desk, listened to what I had to say and made lots of notes. I told her about my smile, my skin, my eating disorder and how it changed my behaviour and my relationship with my family and friends, and I also talked to her about my issues of not having a boyfriend and that on the one hand I wanted to have a boyfriend so much, but on the other hand I was afraid of letting anyone close to me and letting anyone touch me. When I started talking about the boyfriend issue, she asked me if I have sex. I said no. I was surprised about her asking this question and felt somewhat uncomfortable. She asked me why I don't have sex. I said I don't because I don't have a boyfriend. She meant it feels good and that I would like it and that I should think about having it. I did not like her asking these questions and making these comments. What did it matter to her if I slept with someone or not? I was not here to talk about this; I was here to figure out my life to get healthy again. I found her comments rude and inappropriate, and I was offended. At the end of the session, she gave me a business card of another specialist and told me to call him. She said I was 'too advanced' for her, 'too deep in my eating disorder that she could not help me anymore'. After she said that, the appointment was over.

I left her office and was totally confused. I did not know what to think. I felt discouraged and like a hopeless case. I never called the other therapist; I did not want to waste any more money on a doctor just to hear that "I am too messed up to get help".

For the next two years I continued my self-destructive path of bulimia. But no matter how much food I ate, I was not able to fill the emptiness that I felt inside of me. I wasted so much money on food; I don't even want to think about the amount I spent on my binges. I withdrew even more socially than I did before. I spent most of my time alone – either eating or trying to get rid of what I had eaten. I lead a lonely and sad life and I had little hope about ever getting better. I spent so much time in my room, alone, escaping in the virtual computer world. Here I was safe, nobody was able to see me, to judge me or hurt me. I know my parents were very worried about me, but they had no idea how to get close to me. And when they tried, it was not successful – I did not let anyone get close to me. I completely shut off. I cried almost every day, sometimes even a couple of times a day. What had happened to me? How could I let it come that far? I felt completely hopeless. I wanted to get better and be happy and healthy again... but I did not even know where to start my journey towards recovery. Besides, I was not even sure if there was such a thing as 'recovery'...

Just looking at myself in the mirror made me cry. I hated my face, my body, everything. There was nothing pretty about me. Even though, my skin had improved and got really nice over time and I stopped wearing make up to cover up my face, I did not recognize this or was grateful for it. Even though my acne was gone, it still did not change the fact that I hated my face – and my smile.

My turning point was when I met a wonderful man from Canada who is now my husband. I was 21 years old. We met in London and it was love at first sight. We immediately had a special bond between us and it seemed as if we had known one another for a long time already. It almost felt like 'coming home'. It felt wonderful to be close to him. I felt safe. He was also my first boyfriend. I finally had what I was longing for for so long --- a loving, caring and understanding man by my side, who truly and deeply loved me.

In the beginning, I didn't tell him about my eating disorder. I was afraid that if he found out he would leave me. And I did not want him to leave me. I was afraid of being alone and all by myself again. When I was around him, I would eat "normal" and it felt good. For the first time in years I felt "normal". I decided to move to Canada with him and we moved together very quickly, which in the long run really helped me with my eating disorder.

With moving to Canada, a dream of mine also came true. For years I had had the desire to move abroad and to spend some time in another country. When I was 14 years old, I went to England with two friends for three weeks to improve my poor English. I really enjoyed it there and fell in love with the language. And at that point I decided that I wanted to marry someone who speaks English; I wanted to speak English in my relationship! I just loved the way this language sounded! Over the next couple of years, I sometimes told my friends about this dream of mine – of moving abroad and marrying someone who speaks English. I don't know if they took me seriously or not, but deep inside I was. But this dream did not only have to do with the language…. Over the years, while struggling with eating disorders, my desire of living abroad became stronger and stronger. I wanted to travel, I wanted to live some place else – some place where they spoke English, though. I thought that with moving away, I would be able to leave all my problems behind and start over – without my eating disorder! I thought I would finally be free! I would be happy.

But I could not have been more wrong… I was so looking forward to moving to Canada, to start over, to create a 'better' life – I had so many plans… BUT… Nothing had changed. Running away from my problems did not work. And why should it have? I cannot run away from them, and I never would be able to because the real 'problem' was ME.

I still binged but I was not able to do it as often anymore because I would only binge when I was alone and since Brandon and I lived together, we spent a lot of time together. He never noticed my binges but he noticed that I had stomach aches on a regular basis and he was worried about me. I always told him I have problems adjusting to the food here in Canada and that is where my stomach aches came from. He never doubted what I said and never acted suspicious. He also had no reason to – why would I lie to him? But I did lie to him, and I lied a lot. I felt like I had to, as if I had no other choice. I did not want him to find out what was really going on with me. I was afraid of losing him, of being left alone.

It took almost a year till I was ready to tell him about what was going on with me. He hadn't even noticed and I think he was quite surprised about it. He took me in his arms, gave me a kiss and said that we would get through this together and that he would always be there for me and do whatever it took to get me healthy again. I started crying. It felt like a heavy weight had been lifted of my shoulders. Brandon believed in me, in us, and that together we would be able to beat this disorder. For the first time in years, I felt that maybe recovery was possible for me...

And today, I am healthy. I am grateful for my body and love myself and my life. And I am thankful that my body has not given up on me after many years of abuse.

My journey to recovery was difficult at times and I had to take one day after the other. I had setbacks, I had a lot. And every time I fell, I got up again and continued on my journey. I did my best not to look back but forward. Brandon was always there for me and with me, every step of the way. We talked a lot and I told him everything, and I mean EVERYTHING. There were a lot of things I told him that were not pretty, but no matter what I said; his feelings for me did not get any less. He never judged me or my behaviour, no matter what I did. The only thing he did not want me to do was to lie to him and cover up things. It was important for him that I always told him the truth – no matter how 'bad' it was. This was one of the hardest patterns for me to break – to stop lying. I had been lying about my eating behaviour for so many years; I did not even notice it any more when I did... it just happened automatically.

My husband also taught me to smile again. He always told me I looked pretty when I smiled and that I am a beautiful girl. I did not believe him at first... but over time I was able to see that I was a beautiful girl, inside and out, with a beautiful smile. Now, I actually love my smile. I did not smile on pictures for almost ten years, and now, whenever pictures are taken I am the first one to smile!

I am so thankful for having Brandon in my life. He was always there for me; he always believed in me and never gave up on me. His love and support were what I needed to find the strength in me to beat this disorder.

I have reached the point where I am able to openly and honestly talk about my eating disorder struggles and everything connected with it. I am not ashamed anymore of my past and don't feel the need to hide it anymore. I always saw my eating disorder as something negative, as somewhat 'lost years'. And now, for the first time, I can see it in a positive way. If it was not for my past, I know I would not be who I am today and I would not be where I am today --- and I like the person that I am today and I love my life. I very strongly believe that everything happens for a reason, even though many times we are not able to see this reason right away. While I was struggling, I often asked myself what good reason all this pain, all these tears could possible have, and I never found an answer. Now, for the first time, things start to fall in place and make sense. All this was a big learning experience for me – a learning experience that was necessary to make me to the person I am today. It was a painful and difficult experience, that is for sure, but it was necessary for me to get to where I am today. I have learnt so much over the past couple of years, about life and about myself, which I would not have learned otherwise. I know now who I am. I have found my place in life; I have found my personal meaning of my life.

My life is not about myself anymore. For years I was a lonely and depressed girl who lived a small and sad life. Now, I have the desire to make a difference in other people's lives and want to give back to society. It is my passion to show other individuals struggling with eating disorders that there is a way out of this and that these disorders can be beaten. I am in the process of setting up a non-profit eating disorder organization which raises eating disorder awareness and also provides support for individuals struggling with these disorders.

I want you to know that it **IS** possible to recover. **Please don't give up on yourself. You can get through this!** I know. I did it, and so can you! Your eating disorder didn't just happen overnight, it started a long time ago before you first binged, purged or starved yourself – it will take time to get better. One step at a time. Eating disorders are not simply about food and weight but are an attempt to use food and weight to deal with emotional problems. Eating disorders are just the symptoms of something deeper going on inside. Food and your body are not the enemy, even though it sometimes feels like it. You can learn to enjoy your life again. Please keep on believing in yourself and continue to be strong.

You are a wonderful human being - one day, I know, you will be able to see it!

All the best from my heart,

Andrea

By Andrea Roe, 24, Austrian. Married to a wonderful Canadian. Currently living in Langley, British Columbia, Canada. Anorexia for 2 years. Bulimia for 4 years. Depression. Recovered. For more information, please go to **www.eating-disorder-information.com** or send an e-mail to **andrea@eating-disorder-information.com**.

Supporting Survivors of Sexual Abuse and Rape

Supporting Survivors of Sexual Abuse and Rape

Over the course of putting together this book, I spent a good amount of time finding out how people developed their eating disorders. Among other causes, I noticed that people who had endured sexual abuse had a much higher risk of developing eating disorders due to underlying body image negativity and low self esteem. Sufferers of sexual abuse often develop 'coping mechanisms' in order to survive the painful memories of the abuse. Eating disorders are among these mechanisms – but are a very destructive way of coping.

It is shocking that these crimes are not more talked about in our society since it is such a wide spread problem all over the world. Sexual abuse does not discriminate when choosing its victims. It can happen to anyone.

If you or someone you know has been sexually abused – please speak out, seek help and get support. Your silence does not heal you or make your pain go away! Discussing sexual abuse is not easy but it is important to talk about this and to break the silence. You do not have to keep your secret hidden anymore! I want you to understand that it was NOT your fault, you did nothing wrong and did not deserve this! I encourage you to speak out, ask for help and to start your healing journey today! It IS possible to heal the wounds!

While putting together this book, I got in touch with a wonderful woman from Australia named Whitedove. She is a childhood sexual abuse survivor herself and in the following pages you will find her personal story, a poem and a short story written by her. Whitedove also created a website called www.whitedovesnest.com which is a site dedicated to survivors of sexual abuse and those that support them.

There are online communities to support, empower and educate survivors of sexual abuse and rape. You can anonymously share your story, feelings, and fears and get in touch with other individuals who have similar experiences and emotions. At the back of the book you will find some website addresses for more information and support on sexual abuse and rape. Please have a look at them!

Please remember, you are NOT alone! There are others out there just like you.

Whitedove's Story

By Whitedove, Australia. Childhood Sexual Abuse Survivor. 8 years into my Healing Journey.

My name is Whitedove and I was sexually abused by my father for six years. Though this is a simple sentence, for me, it has basically ruled my life since I was around 11 years old. Two elder sisters and a childhood friend were abused by him as well.

I started dealing with the abuse in 1998, when I went to a counselor for what I deemed at the time as relationship issues with my then boyfriend, and I started to want to deal with why I was so unhappy and depressed. I attended this counselor for a number of years, weekly at times, monthly at others, to help me through. It was tough work, very emotionally draining and at times extremely frightening. I continued to seek help in whatever way I could.

I joined a sexual abuse recovery group in 2000 where I was helped out by other women in similar situations to my own. It was through lots of counseling, helping hands from my husband and friends, that I was able to confront my father in 2000. It was a difficult time, and very daunting, but I could not continue on with the fallacies and lies that I was living with while visiting my family.

The confrontation was awful, but I gained a sense of purpose and understanding from it. I realized that I was not at fault and that I could speak up and confront the person who I had feared for all those years. I no longer have a relationship with either my mother or my father. They are both still alive, and my mother still lives with him, even though he admits he abused three of his daughters.

My other two sisters are in denial, and it makes it hard. I have had to step in twice now when their children have been put in harms way. I do not want to risk other children being harmed by this man. Unfortunately my sisters do not agree with my stance and are still visiting the abuser, knowing their own stories and my own. I hope one day that they can realize what has happened, and to begin to heal from our childhood.

It has come to the point now where I have lost all of my immediate family, because I find it too difficult to visit them, knowing that there is this between us all, and nothing is said. I feel like I have to live a lie when I am around them. I have sought out other relationships where I feel I can be supported and understood.

When I first started dealing with the abuse, I did not know what it had done to me emotionally, and it was not until I examined my life and my childhood that I started to realize that my childhood was not "normal". At the time, I felt completely alone with this issue, thought that only I had been abused in the family and felt that I was completely at fault, somehow explaining to myself that the abuse "did not really matter" in the whole scheme of things.

How wrong I was. I had extremely low self esteem, constantly blamed myself and degraded myself, had suicidal thoughts, fought boughts of depression, shaking and anxiety, sickness and migraines. It was not until I started to deal with the abuse issue, that I realized how it had affected me

I now live a completely different life. I am generally happier and calmer and have more of an understanding of who I am, and where I have come from. I recommend to anyone who is considering counseling for this issue, to stick with it, read books, listen to yourself, talk to people who you can trust and know that **you are not alone**. I have created the site www.whitedovesnest.com to help others write their story, so they can shout out loud on the web their experiences. Please feel free to visit the site. It is completely anonymous.

By Whitedove, Australia. Childhood Sexual Abuse Survivor. 8 years into my Healing Journey. For more information on sexual abuse, go to **www. whitedovesnest.com** – a site dedicated to survivors of sexual abuse and those that support them. This website provides information on sexual abuse, personal stories, articles, inspiration and help to those affected by sexual abuse, rape and molestation.

LITTLE GIRL GONE

by Whitedove

The winter wind blows against my face
The tear weeps, it leaves no trace
My heart expands when I see you gone
It is for you that I will ever mourn

That little girl I once used to be
The quiet girl that was me
Has disappeared, and I cry a tear
Forever in my heart; forever near

I look at photos now many years on
I see the look that is now gone
The tears of sorrow, downward gaze
The darkened avenues; the grey haze

For now I fit another mould
I see rainbows and pots of gold
I look up and see a bright blue sky
I see happiness standing by

The time for joy is here at last
It is here, it comes so fast
The smile of love shows its face
A greatness now in sorrow's place.

THE OWL AND THE EAGLE

by Whitedove

The wise old owl sat in the canopy of the forest, gazing across the calm plains and ocean. She was content in her wishes, which grew from her experience and knowledge. She glanced down and noticed a baby eagle, hunched on the forest floor, crying.

"Why eagle do you cry?" asked the owl.

"I am lost and all alone," replied the eagle.

"Fly, fly up here to the canopy, see the ocean that lives beyond," said the owl.

"There is no ocean, and I cannot fly, the forest is too dark and my wings too small" said the baby eagle, now crying more, tears silently slipping down to the forest floor.

With this, the owl circled down from her resting place, landing just above where the eagle sat. Her face held a smile of wisdom.

"Though you cannot see it now, the ocean is there, and there is a light that surrounds the forest that is dazzling. They call this light love – little eagle."

"But what is love?" cried the eagle.

"Love is what makes us fly and see what is beyond our boundaries"

Though it took the eagle time, and patience, the eagle learnt to fly, and you can now see her circling high above the clouds basking in the light of the sun, whispering to others, what the wise old owl once told her.

List of Contributors

In Alphabetical order:

Amanda Travers Bell, 21, married. Nashville, Tennessee, United States. Anorexia, Bulimia, and Binge Eating for 8 years. Depression, Self-Mutilation, Codependency, Cocaine Addiction, Survivor of Rape and Abuse. In Recovery for over 2 years, and getting stronger everyday!

Andrea Roe, 24, Austrian. Married to a wonderful Canadian. Currently living in Langley, British Columbia, Canada. Anorexia for 2 years. Bulimia for 4 years. Depression. Recovered. For more information, go to **www.eating-disorder-information.com** or send an e-mail to **andrea@eating-disorder-information.com**.

Angela C., 19. Pennsylvania, USA. Bulimia. Anxiety and Depression. In Strong Recovery.

Anita Humphries, 26, engaged. Birmingham, United Kingdom. Anorexia for 2 years and Bulimia for 8 years. Sexual Abuse. Self-Harm. Depression and Social Anxiety. Recovered.

Anna Paterson, 37. England. Engaged to Simon Teff. Author of eating disorder recovery books. Anorexia for 14 years. Sexual, Emotional and Physical Abuse Survivor. Self-Harm. Recovered. For more information, visit Anna's website at **www.annapaterson.com** or send an e-mail to **Anna@anorectic.fsnet.co.uk**

Christina, 24. The Netherlands. Struggling with an Eating Disorder for 7 years. In Recovery. For more information, visit Christina's **website at www.geocities. com/spacey_christina/**

Emma McClelland, 18. Manchester, England. Anorexia for 2 years, turned Bulimia for 1 year. Self-Harm. Recovered.

Geri Karlstrom, 53. Surrey, British Columbia, Canada. Recovering for over 40 years from an Eating Disorder. Expressing herself through music has helped Geri through her recovery from an eating disorder. If you suffer from eating disorders, abuse, depression or addiction issues, this music is just for you. Geri's music has touched people from all over the world. For more information, go to **www.geri. net.**

Izayana, 23. Mexico. Anorexia for 12 years. Depression. Self-Harm. Recovered.

Jamie Walker, 31. Nebraska, United States. Battling an Eating Disorder and Depression for 13 years. In Recovery. Planning to go back to school later this year and finish getting her Human Services degree.

Jessica, 26. Houston, Texas, USA. Suffered from COE (Compulsive Overeating) turned Anorexia turned Bulimia turned EDNOS (Eating Disorder Not Otherwise Specified) - total of 12 and a half years. 7 time Relapse-Survivor (from the year 2000 to 2005). Finally Fully Recovered! Childhood Sexual Abuse and Rape Survivor. Recovered Cutter. Diagnosed with Mental Illness. Symptom Free from Mental Illness for 1 year! If you want to get in touch with Jessica, please send an e-mail to **ribbons_undone@sbcglobal.net.**

Jessica Beal, 20. United States. Binge Purge Anorexia for 4 years. Self-Harm. Recovered. For more information, visit Jessica's website "One Life – Sharing, the Key to Hope" at **http://river-tree.net/onelife/**

Julie Ramirez, 35. United States. Bulimia for 10 years. In Recovery.

Kate Holden, 20. London, England. Anorexia from age 13. Self-Harm. Recovered. Teaching Assistant and part-time photography student, starting Midwifery degree in September 2006.

Katherine Roemer, 19. Kentucky, USA. 7 years with EDNOS (Eating Disorder Not Otherwise Specified) and Anorexia. Sexual Assault and Abuse Survivor. Self-Harm. Recently Declared Recovered.

Kim Ratcliffe, 44. British Columbia, Canada. Anorexia on and off for over 20 years. 12 years Recovery. For more information on Kim's personal journey and her journal writings, go to **http://www.angelfire.com/oh3/anorexia** or send an email to **kvrat@shaw.ca.**

Krystal Malisheske, 18. Sartell, Minnesota, United States. Bulimia and Anorexia for 2 years. Recovered.

LA Crompton, 37, married, two children. New York, USA. Anorexia/Bulimia 10 years. Recovered 12 years. For more information, go to **www.dreamer-girl.com.**

Laurie Daily. San Diego, California, USA. Recovered 14 years from all Eating Disorders. Laurie is a professional singer and Certified Eating Disorder Specialist who has dedicated her music to eating disorder recovery. All of the songs on Laurie's CDs relate to her own journey from eating disorders to heal in hopes to inspire others to live a life free from anorexia, bulimia, and compulsive eating. For more information, go to **www.lauriedaily.com** and **www.harmony-grove.com.**

Lisa Horsfield, 32. New Zealand. Bulimia for 10 years. In Recovery for 9 years.

Lori Henry, 24. Vancouver, British Columbia, Canada. Bulimic for 5 years. Recovered. Author of "Silent Screams", a collection of poems at the core of her journey in recovering from bulimia. For more information, go to **www.trafford. com/robots/02-0694.html** and **http://eatingdisorders.suite101.com.**

Mara McWilliams, 37. Married with a ten year old daughter. California, United States. In recovery with a diagnosis of Bipolar Disorder, Panic Disorder, and Anorexia. Mara is an artist and expresses herself through painting and poetry. The freedom and release she finds in painting has been nearly as beneficial to her recovery as therapy. Mara's ultimate goal is to educate our society that through proper diagnosis, treatment, therapy, love, support, and understanding, recovery is possible. Please remember, as with any other illness, educating ourselves about our disorder is extremely important. For more information, go to **www.recovery-throughart.com.**

Michelle, 31. Vancouver, British Columbia, Canada. Restricting and Bingeing for 12 years. Recovered.

Michelle R Wilson, 28, Single. Vancouver, British Columbia, Canada. Anorexia-Bulimia for 10 years. Recovered however still occasionally challenged. Also history of Depression and Social Anxiety. Visual artist, focus on painting people. Currently work with adults with disabilities.

N.C, 30. Canada. Disordered Eating for 6 years. In Recovery. Practicing Mindfulness Meditation Daily.

Nadia Lovell, 29. Wales, England. Anorexia and Bulimia for 12 years. Recovered. I have set up a self help group in Cardiff and am on the path of qualifying as a councillor so I am able to help others who are experiencing the distress of suffering from an eating disorder. If you want to get in touch with Nadia, feel free to send an e-mail to **nadialovell@yahoo.co.uk.**

Rachel Beattie, 25. Taunton, England. Former Anorexic, Bulimic, Self-harmer. Recovered.

Regina Edgar, 20. Michigan, USA. Anorexia and Bulimia for 9 years. Self-Injury for 5 years. Sexual Abuse. In Recovery. Feel free to contact Regina at **youngfiddler@hotmail.com.**

Sarah Kipp, 26. Las Vegas, Nevada, USA. EDNOS (Eating Disorder Not Otherwise Specified) for 14 years. In Strong Recovery. If you want to get in touch with Sarah, feel free to send an e-mail to **slkipp@yahoo.com.**

Shinyflower, 23. Nurse. Norway. Anorexia for 6 years. Recovered. If you want to get in touch with Shinyflower, send an e-mail to **lillebie@europe.com.**

Stephanie, 20. Arizona, USA. Anorexia for 6 years. Self-Harm. Survivor of Sexual Abuse and Rape. Recovered.

Tiffannie Brinkhaus, 25. Minnesota USA. Overeating Disorder brought on by Depression. In Recovery.

Vera Fleischer, 30. Germany. EDNOS (Eating Disorder Not Otherwise Specified) for 2 years. Depression. Diagnosed with Mental Illness and OCD (Obsessive Compulsive Disorder). Recovered. For more information, please go to **www.verabug.com.**

Whitedove, Australia. Childhood Sexual Abuse Survivor. 8 years into my Healing Journey. For more information on sexual abuse, go to **www.whitedovesnest.com** - a site dedicated to survivors of sexual abuse and those that support them. This website provides information on sexual abuse, personal stories, articles, inspiration and help to those affected by sexual abuse, rape and molestation.

Whitney Laree Greenwood Johnson, 18. Multiethnic. Single. Social Service Student. Salem, Oregon, United States. Bulimic but went through an Anorexic stage, Excessive Dieter, for almost 8 years. In Recovery. Have Self Injured on occasion mostly recovered from that. Depression, Anxiety, Panic Disorder, Under Control. Recovered from Suicidal Thoughts, have attempted Suicide. Attention Deficit Hyperactivity Disorder.

Websites on Eating Disorders

Something Fishy

www.somethingfishy.org

Something-Fishy provides information on all forms of Eating Disorders, related topics, plus much more, and most important of all, it provides support to everyone affected by Eating Disorders, and their loved-ones.

Pale Reflections

www.pale-reflections.com

Pale Reflections is an online community for everyone affected by Eating Disorders and provides information on all forms of Eating Disorders, Depression, Obsessive Compulsive Disorder, and much more.

Eating Disorder Referral

www.edreferral.com

EDReferral.com provides information and treatment resources for all forms of eating disorders. This site provides assistance, in the form of information and resources, to those suffering with eating disorders to get them started on the road to recovery and healthy living.

Bulimia.com (Gürze Books)

www.bulimia.com

Bulimia.com specializes in information about eating disorders including Anorexia, Bulimia, and Binge Eating Disorder, plus related topics such as Body Image and Obesity. This website offers eating disorder books at discounted prices, articles about eating disorders, newsletters, and links to treatment facilities, organizations, other websites, and much more.

Websites on Self-Harm

RecoverYourLife.com

www.recoveryourlife.com

RecoverYourLife.com is one of the biggest and best Self-Harm Communities on the Internet. Communicate with other members and realize you are not alone. Whether you want help in reducing or stopping your Self-Harm, or you just aren't ready yet, everyone is welcome here. RecoverYourLife's members have proved many thousands of times that Self-Harm can be beaten and that there is hope.

LifeSIGNS (Self-Injury Guidance & Network Support)

www.selfharm.org

LifeSIGNS is a voluntary organization that raises awareness about the syndrome of self-injury in the UK and beyond. LifeSIGNS provides much needed information and training to organizations; offering unique services not available from any other voluntary organizations.

S.A.F.E. Alternatives (Self-Abuse Finally Ends)

www.safe-alternatives.com or www.selfinjury.com

S.A.F.E. Alternatives (Self-Abuse Finally Ends) is a nationally recognized treatment approach, professional network and educational resource base, which is committed to helping you and others achieve an end to self-injurious behavior.

Young People and Self-Harm

www.selfharm.org.uk

This site is a key information resource for young people who self-harm, their friends and families, and professionals working with them.

Websites on Sexual Abuse and Rape

Broken Spirits

www.brokenspirits.com

Broken Spirits is an online community and support group that focuses on aiding both current and past victims of child abuse, sexual abuse, and domestic violence. This website is an interactive, personal support related website dedicated to helping each other through the pain and fear of an abusive relationship. It provides a comprehensive International Directory of shelters, hotlines and organizations that can provide help for potential victims. In addition to the national abuse resource listing is a comprehensive discussion forum where users can create their own virtual identity within complete confidentiality.

After Silence

www.aftersilence.org

After Silence is a community designed to help survivors communicate in the recovery of rape, and sexual abuse; and to support, empower, validate, and educate survivors of rape and sexual abuse, as well as secondary survivors. The core of this website is a community where survivors come together online in a mutually supportive environment.

Whitedove's Nest

www.whitedovesnest.com

Whitedove's Nest is dedicated to survivors of sexual abuse and those that support them. It provides information on sexual abuse, personal stories, articles, inspiration and help to those affected by sexual abuse, rape and molestation.

The Rape, Abuse & Incest National Network (RAINN)

www.rainn.org

The Rape, Abuse & Incest National Network (RAINN) is the nation's largest anti-sexual assault organization. Among its programs, RAINN created and operates the National Sexual Assault Hotline at 1.800.656.HOPE. This nationwide partner-ship of more than 1,100 local rape treatment hotlines provides victims of sexual assault with free, confidential services around the clock.

Joshua Childrens Foundation

www.joshuachildrensfoundation.org

Joshua Childrens Foundation provides information and links to help in the healing process of victims of sexual child abuse. Whether you are a child or an adult survi-vor of childhood sexual child abuse, you can find helpful sources and suggestions on our website to help in your healing.

ISBN 141209617-0